MR ANGIOGRAPHY:
A Teaching File

MR ANGIOGRAPHY:
A Teaching File

Editors

MICHAEL BRANT-ZAWADZKI, M.D.
Hoag Memorial Hospital
Newport Beach, California

OREST B. BOYKO, M.D.
Department of Radiology
Duke University Medical Center
Durham, North Carolina

MAUREEN C. JENSEN, M.D.
Hoag Memorial Hospital
Newport Beach, California

GARY D. GILLAN, R.T.
Hoag Memorial Hospital
Newport Beach, California

RAVEN PRESS ✒ NEW YORK

Raven Press, Ltd., 1185 Avenue of the Americas, New York, New York 10036

Made in the United States of America

Library of Congress Cataloging-in-Publication Data

MR angiography : a teaching file / editors, Michael Brant-Zawadzki, Orest B.
Boyko, Maureen Jensen.
  p. cm.
 Includes bibliographical references and index.
 ISBN 0-7817-0093-0
 1. Blood-vessels—Magnetic resonance imaging.—Case Studies.
I. Brandt-Zawadzki, Michael. II. Boyko, Orest B. (Orest Bohdan),
1955– . III. Jensen, Maureen.
 [DNLM: 1. Vascular Diseases—diagnosis—case studies. 2. Magnetic
Resonance Imaging—methods. 3. Blood Vessels—pathology.
4. Angiography—methods. WG 500 M939 1993]
RC691.6.A53M75 1993
616.1′607′548—dc20
DNLM/DLC
for Library of Congress   93-16482
                CIP

9 8 7 6 5 4 3 2 1

To my husband, Michael, for his love and
unfailing support, and our children, Kyle and Leah.

M.C. Jensen

Contents

Michael Brant-Zawadzki, M.D., F.A.C.R. *Hoag Memorial Hospital, 301 Newport Blvd., Box Y, Newport Beach, CA 92658*

Orest B. Boyko, M.D., Ph.D. *Department of Radiology, Duke University Medical Center, Box 3808, Durham, NC 27710*

Maureen C. Jensen, M.D. *Hoag Memorial Hospital, 301 Newport Blvd., Box Y, Newport Beach, CA 92658*

Gary D. Gillan, R.T. *Hoag Memorial Hospital, 301 Newport Blvd., Box Y, Newport Beach, CA 92658*

This book is designed to familiarize the resident and practicing radiologist with the current applications of MRA. MRA techniques have been in clinical use only in recent years and have already become a valuable adjunct to routine clinical MRI. Modifications to existing hardware and software are continuously improving the quality of MRA and expanding MRI's role in evaluation of vascular disease. Most of the commonly encountered vascular lesions amenable to depiction by MRA are illustrated. In addition, we have included artifacts that can lead to interpretive errors. The reader is encouraged to review the key images and history on the left-hand page prior to reading the diagnosis and discussion on the right-hand page. The references at the end of each case are provided for more in-depth discussion for the interested reader.

Michael Brant-Zawadzki, M.D.
Orest B. Boyko, M.D.
Maureen C. Jensen, M.D.
Gary D. Gillan, R.T.

Acknowledgments

At Hoag, we sincerely thank Janet Arnds for her countless hours of manuscript preparation, Cheryl Kosky for medical photography, and technologists Jim Walling, Randi Burns, Debbie Norman, Sonia Halter, Mike Thomas, and Jackie Oldeck for case procurement.

Michael Brant-Zawadzki, M.D.
Maureen C. Jensen, M.D.
Gary D. Gillan, R.T.

MR ANGIOGRAPHY:
A Teaching File

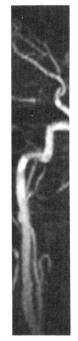

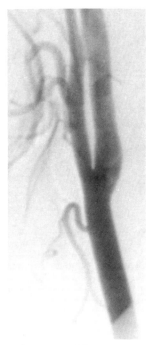

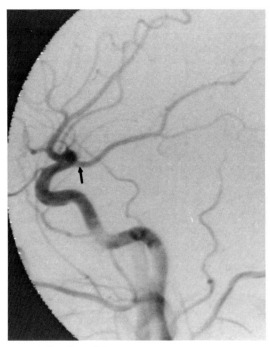

FIG. 1A. LCCA
2D TOF MRA.

FIG. 1B. LCCA conven-
tional angiogram.

FIG. 1C. LICA conventional angiogram.

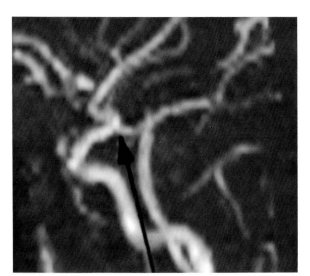

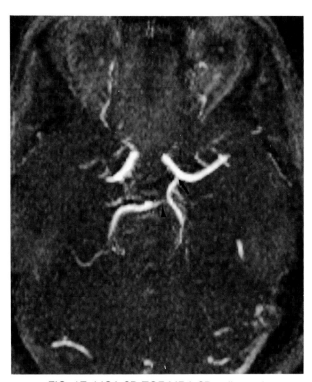

FIG. 1D. LICA 2D TOF MRA 3D reprojection.

FIG. 1E. LICA 2D TOF MRA 2D collapsed.

Clinical History

Magnetic resonance angiography in 17-, 74-, 59-, and 66-year-old patients.

Findings

Two-dimensional (2D) time-of-flight (TOF) magnetic resonance angiography (MRA) (Fig. 1A) and conventional angiography (Fig. 1B) demonstrate a normal carotid bulb of the left common carotid artery (LCCA) in a 17-year-old. The left internal carotid artery (LICA) conventional angiogram shows a fetal origin of the left posterior cerebral artery (PCA) (Fig. 1C, *arrow*); shown also on 2D TOF MRA 3D reprojection (Fig. 1D, *arrow*) and 2D collapsed (Fig. 1E, *arrow*) images. Note the hypoplastic P1 segment (Fig. 1E, *arrowhead*).

T2-weighted MR image in a 74-year-old shows normal flow void in the bilateral posterior communicating arteries (PCoA) (Fig. 1F, *arrows*) visualized better on 2D TOF (Fig. 1G, *right arrows*) than on 3D TOF (Fig. 1G, *left*). Note the better saturation of stationary protons (brain and fat) on the 2D TOF than on the 3D TOF MRA (Fig. 1G).

The 2D phase contrast (PC) MRA in a 59-year-old shows normal direction information of arteries and veins on phase images. In relation to flow relative to right to left gradients the signal intensity in the right internal carotid artery (RICA) is bright and dark in the LICA (Fig. 1H). The flow in the right transverse sinus (RTS) is dark (left to right flow) and bright in the LTS (Fig. 1H).

The 2D PC MRA in a 66-year-old shows differences in signal intensity of intracranial arteries and veins related only to a different choice in velocity encoding (VENC) (200 cm/sec left image in Fig. 1I and 80 cm/sec right image in Fig. 1I). The slower flow of the transverse sinuses is better seen at the lower VENC.

Diagnosis

Normal MRA flow and anatomy.

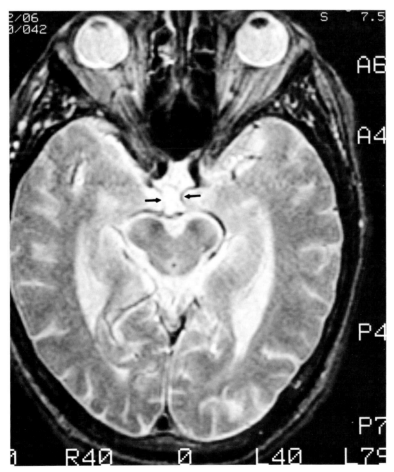

FIG. 1F. SE 2117/80.

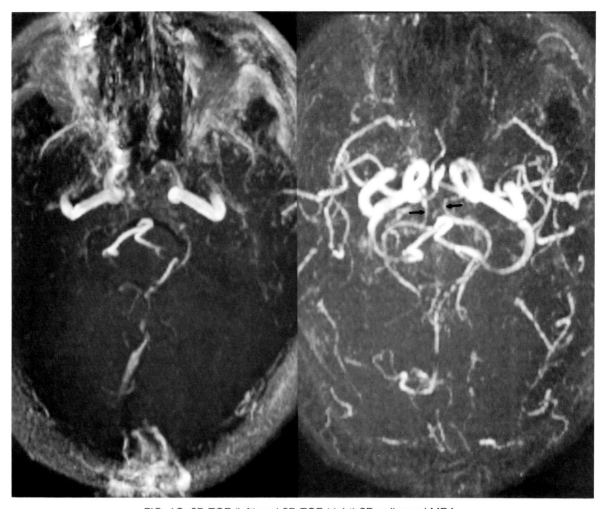

FIG. 1G. 3D TOF (left) and 2D TOF (right) 2D collapsed MRA.

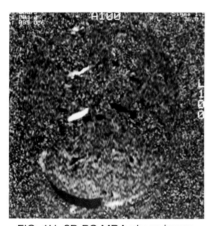

FIG. 1H. 2D PC MRA phase image.

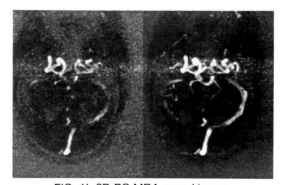

FIG. 1I. 2D PC MRA speed image.

Discussion

It is important to keep in mind, however, that MRA image optimization can be equipment dependent. For example, time-of-flight image quality varies with manufacturer pulse sequence design. Additionally, phase contrast technique is not yet available on all equipment. The availability of a variety of MRA pulse sequence acquisitions gives numerous options for optimal vascular imaging (1).

Reference

1. Turski P, Bernstein M, Boyko O, et al. *Vascular magnetic resonance imaging,* vol 3. GE Medical Systems Application Guide, Milwaukee, WI, 1990.

Submitted by: Orest B. Boyko, M.D., Ph.D., Duke University Medical Center, Durham, North Carolina; Michael Brant-Zawadzki, M.D., F.A.C.R., Senior Editor.

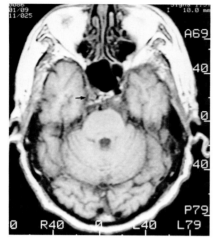

FIG. 2A. SE 500/20.

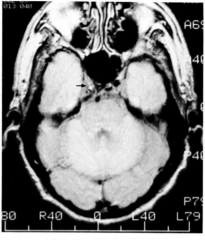

FIG. 2B. SE 2100/30.

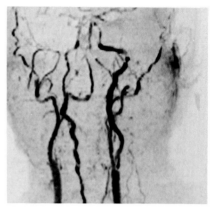

FIG. 2C. 2D TOF MRA 45/9.

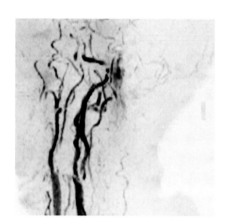

FIG. 2D. 2D TOF MRA, 45/9.

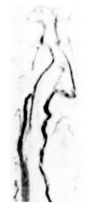

FIG. 2E. 2D TOF MRA, 45/9, selective masking RICA.

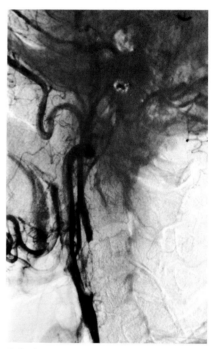

FIG. 2F. Conventional RICA angiogram.

Clinical History

A 76-year-old male with transient ischemic attacks (TIAs).

Findings

There is a lack of normal flow void in the right internal carotid artery (RICA) on both T1- and T2-weighted images (Figs. 2A and B, *arrows*). No infarcts are seen.

The 2D time-of-flight (TOF) magnetic resonance angiogram (MRA) (Figs. 2C and D) shows high-grade stenosis of the RICA, but presence of flow in the petrous and supraclinoid portion of the RICA. Also, stenosis of the left arterial carotid origin is present. Selective masking and reprojection of the right carotid better demonstrates the critical stenosis (Fig. 2E) seen as a discontinuity of flow-related enhancement in the vessel. Conventional angiography demonstrates the critical RICA stenosis (Fig. 2F) and filling of the intracranial portion of the RICA retrograde through the ophthalmic artery (Fig. 2G) and antegrade (Fig. 2H) flow through the ICA.

Diagnosis

Severe carotid stenoses from atherosclerotic disease.

Discussion

Loss of normal intracranial arterial flow void at the level of the siphon on conventional spin-echo images can have numerous explanations (1). One consideration is extracranial arterial disease (2) such as illustrated by this case. Although thrombosis and complete occlusion causing loss of flow void can be considered, slow flow or retrograde flow can mimic thrombosis; thus, the value of a flow-sensitive MRA technique is key to patient management.

References

1. Bradley WG. Flow phenomena in MR imaging. *AJR* 1988;150:983–984.
2. Heinz ER, Yeates AE, Djang WT. Significant extracranial carotid stenosis: detection on routine cerebral MR images. *Radiology* 1989;170:843–849.

Submitted by: Orest B. Boyko, M.D., Ph.D., Duke University Medical Center, Durham, North Carolina; Michael Brant-Zawadzki, M.D., F.A.C.R., Senior Editor.

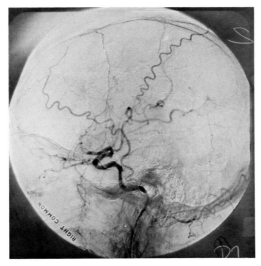

FIG. 2G. Conventional RICA angiogram.

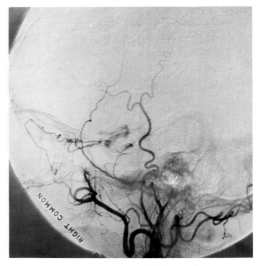

FIG. 2H. Conventional RICA angiogram.

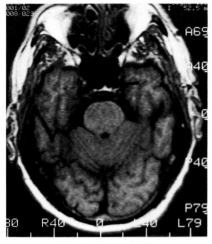
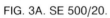

FIG. 3A. SE 500/20.

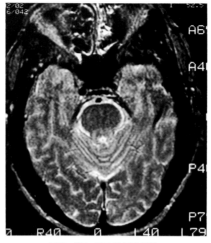

FIG. 3B. SE 2100/80.

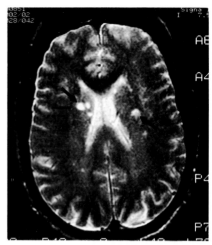

FIG. 3C. SE 2100/80.

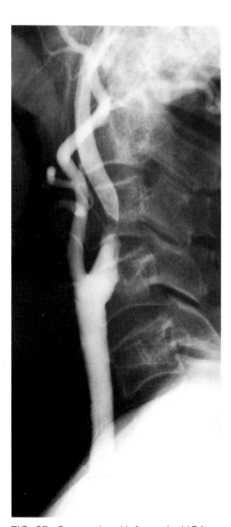

FIG. 3D. Conventional left cervical ICA angiogram.

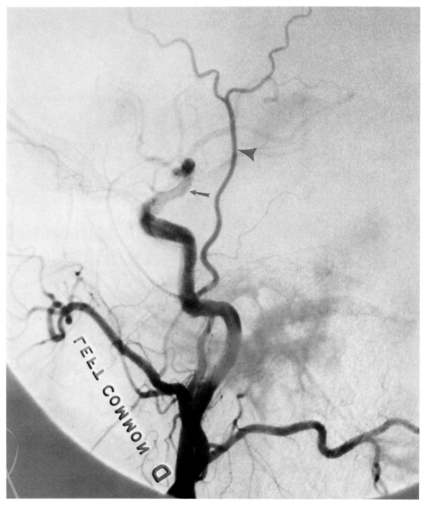

FIG. 3E. Conventional left CCA angiogram.

Clinical History

A 64-year-old male with transient left hemiparesis.

Findings

T1-weighted (Fig. 3A) and T2-weighted (Fig. 3B) images demonstrate equivocally decreased luminal caliber of the left cavernous internal carotid artery (CICA) compared to the right. (Fig. 3A, *arrow*). Bilateral periventricular hyperintensities representing areas of ischemia or infarct are seen or higher convexity T2-weighted image (Fig. 3C, *arrows*). Left common carotid artery (CCA) angiogram shows a high-grade critical stenosis of the proximal ICA (Fig. 3D).

Diagnosis

Severe atherosclerotic stenosis of the left ICA.

Discussion

This case illustrates that the presence of a significant cervical carotid artery stenosis can be accompanied by the presence of normal flow void (1) but there can be an associated decreased vessel diameter due to a decreased pressure gradient and flow distal to the stenosis. On conventional angiography intracranial filling of the external carotid artery branches (Fig. 3E, *arrowhead*) occurs simultaneously with that of the ICA (Fig. 3E, *arrow*), which indicates a reequilibration of flow and a decreased flow in the ICA distal to the stenosis.

Reference

1. Brant-Zawadzki ML. Routine MR imaging of the internal carotid artery siphon: angiographic correlation with cervical carotid lesions. *AJNR* 1990;11:467–471.

Submitted by: Orest B. Boyko, M.D., Ph.D., Duke University Medical Center, Durham, North Carolina; Michael Brant-Zawadzki, M.D., F.A.C.R., Senior Editor.

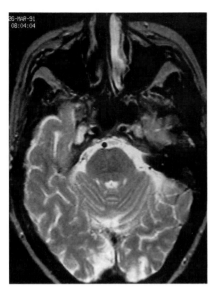

FIG. 4A. Axial SE 2500/90.

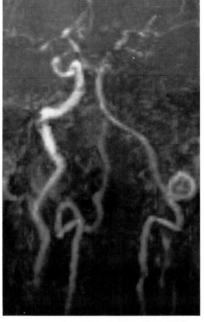

FIG. 4B. 3D TOF (FISP) 40/7/15°.

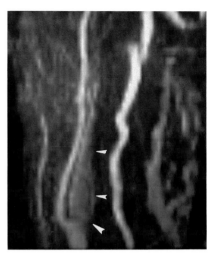

FIG. 4C. 2D TOF (FLASH) 36/10/30°.

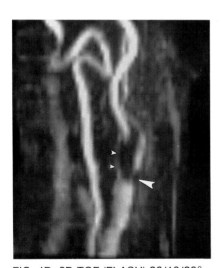

FIG. 4D. 2D TOF (FLASH) 36/10/30°.

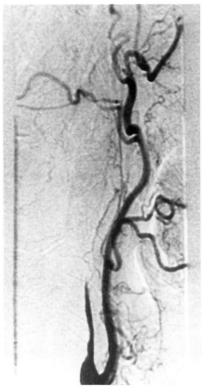

FIG. 4E. Intraarterial DSA LCA injection.

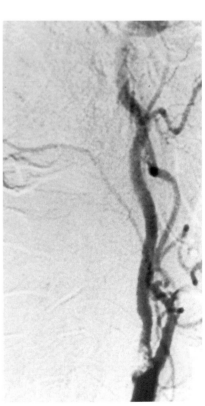

FIG. 4F. Intraarterial DSA RCA injection.

Clinical History

An 87-year-old female with headaches, fainting spells, and transient ischemic attacks (TIAs) in the left carotid distribution.

Findings

The T2-weighted axial MR study (Fig. 4A) demonstrates normal appearance of the carotid arteries at the level of the cavernous sinus level. No distal abnormalities were visualized. The 3D time-of-flight (TOF) magnetic resonance angiogram (MRA) suggests complete occlusion of the left carotid artery (Fig. 4B). Maximum intensity pixel reformations of the left carotid artery with 2D TOF technique (Fig. 4C) suggests the presence of very slow flow in its proximal segment only (*arrowheads*). The contralateral carotid (Fig. 4D) is shown to contain a significant occlusive lesion encircling the origins of both internal (*small arrowheads*) and external (*large arrowhead*) carotid artery origins.

Diagnosis

Recent occlusion of left internal carotid artery with severe stenosis of the right carotid system.

Discussion

The intraarterial angiogram (Fig. 4E) verifies the MR angiographic impression. The left internal carotid artery shows layering of contrast in its very proximal segment with absence of contrast flow distally. The right carotid angiogram does show a plaque, which severely constricts the origin of the internal carotid artery but not the external (Fig. 4F). The intracranial views from the right carotid artery injection (Fig. 4G) shows it supplies both the right and left anterior intracerebral circulations. The tendency for MRA to exaggerate the stenosis with occlusive disease is again demonstrated with regard to the right external carotid artery, when comparing Fig. 4D with Fig. 4F. Also, the level of certainty regarding the complete occlusion of the left carotid is much greater with the intraarterial angiographic study. Of interest, although the carotid siphons are shown on the original MR image (Fig. 4A), the left carotid artery siphon is not well seen with the right carotid artery injection. However, evaluation of the left carotid injection (Fig. 4H) demonstrates a very prominent ophthalmic collateral (*arrow*) indicating that flow into the left carotid artery siphon is through a retrograde ophthalmic route. This would explain the flow void in the left carotid siphon. Again, the detailed anatomic information provided by intraarterial angiograms is somewhat more convincing than that obtained from MRA alone.

References

1. Masaryk AM, Ross JS, et al. 3DFT MR angiography of the carotid bifurcation: potential and limitations as a screening examination. *Radiology* 1991;179:797–804.
2. Heiserman JE, Drayer BP, et al. Carotid artery stenosis: clinical efficacy of two-dimensional time-of-flight MR angiography. *Radiology* 1992;182:761–768.
3. Keller PJ, Drayer BP, et al. MR angiography with two-dimensional acquisition and three-dimensional display. *Radiology* 1989;173:157–532.

Submitted by: Michael Brant-Zawadzki, M.D., F.A.C.R., Hoag Memorial Hospital, Newport Beach, California; Michael Brant-Zawadzki, M.D., F.A.C.R., Senior Editor.

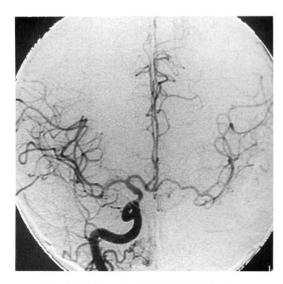

FIG. 4G. Intraarterial DSA RCA injection.

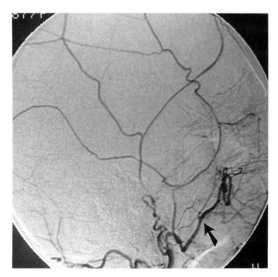

FIG. 4H. Intraarterial DSA LCA injection.

11

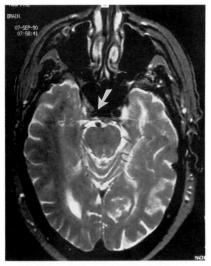

FIG. 5A. Axial SE 2800/90.

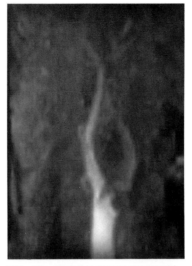

FIG. 5B. 3D TOF (FISP) 30/7/20°.

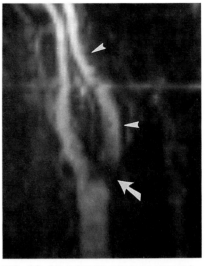

FIG. 5C. 2D TOF (FLASH) 31/10/40°.

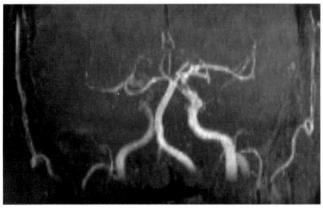

FIG. 5D. 3D TOF (FISP) 50/7/15°.

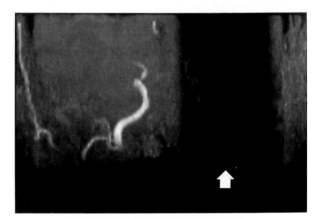

FIG. 5E. 3D TOF (FISP) 50/7/15°.

Clinical History

An 80-year-old male with transient left hemiparesis.

Findings

T2-weighted axial image (Fig. 5A) demonstrates asymmetry of signal in the carotid artery siphons, the right is increased (*arrow*) compared to the normal signal void on the left. The 3D time-of-flight magnetic resonance angiogram (MRA) (maximum intensity pixel reconstruction) of the right common carotid bifurcation (Fig. 5B) shows the external carotid artery well. The internal carotid artery is seen only as a wisp of increased signal intensity, possibly suggesting occlusion. The 2D time-of-flight study (Fig. 5C) obtained immediately after the 3D study demonstrates that the internal carotid artery (*arrowheads*) is not occluded, but does show significantly diminished signal immediately beyond its origin off the common carotid artery. In fact, a complete signal void is apparent (*arrow*). Intracranial MRA (Fig. 5D) shows the diminished flow in the right middle cerebral artery compared with the normal left. Also note that the signal intensity within the right carotid artery is reduced.

Repeat 3D time-of-flight study with spatial saturation (Fig. 5E, *arrow*) of the left carotid artery shows markedly diminished flow in the right middle cerebral branch, demonstrating its predominant supply from collateral flow via the circle of Willis.

Diagnosis

Preocclusive, high-grade stenosis of right internal carotid artery with right middle cerebral artery flow supplied predominantly through the left anterior circulation.

Discussion

The intraarterial angiogram (Fig. 5F) verifies the very severe stenosis of the right internal carotid artery. Intracranial views (Fig. 5G) demonstrate essentially no flow of contrast beyond the carotid siphon. The left carotid artery injection (Fig. 5H) demonstrates cross-flow from the left carotid to the right anterior circulation. This case illustrates the essential problems in defining complete occlusion versus severe stenosis of a carotid artery with MR angiography, particularly when using a 3D technique, as the 2D technique is much more sensitive to slow flow. Note the value of using saturation pulses with the time-of-flight angiographic technique for determining flow contribution.

References

1. Keller PJ, Drayer BP, et al. MR angiography with two-dimensional acquisition and three-dimensional display: work in progress. *Radiology* 1989;173:527–532.
2. Masaryk AM, Ross JS, et al. 3DFT MR angiography of the carotid bifurcation: potential and limitations as a screening examination. *Radiology* 1991;179:797–804.
3. Edelman RR, Mattle HP, et al. Magnetic resonance imaging of flow dynamics in the circle of Willis. *Stroke* 1990;21:56–65.
4. Felmlee LP, Ehman RL. Spatial presaturation: a method for suppressing flow artifacts and improving depiction of vascular anatomy in MR imaging. *Radiology* 1987;164:559–564.

Submitted by: Michael Brant-Zawadzki, M.D., F.A.C.R., Hoag Memorial Hospital, Newport Beach, California; Michael Brant-Zawadzki, M.D., F.A.C.R., Senior Editor.

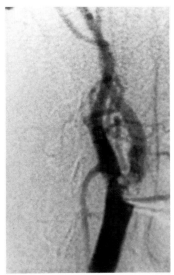

FIG. 5F. Intraarterial DSA RCA.

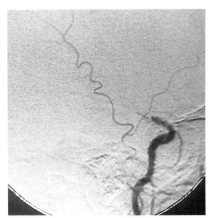

FIG. 5G. Intraarterial DSA RICA.

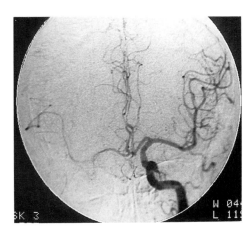

FIG. 5H. Intraarterial DSA LICA.

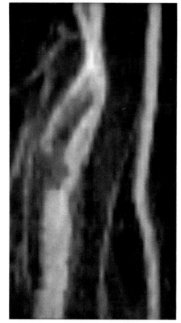

FIG. 6A. 2D TOF (FLASH) 36/10/30°.

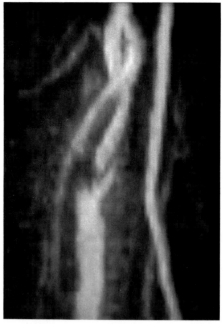

FIG. 6B. 2D TOF (FLASH) 36/10/30°.

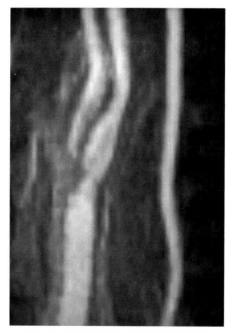

FIG. 6C. 2D TOF (FLASH) 36/10/30°.

Clinical History

A 59-year-old male with right-sided transient ischemic attacks (TIAs).

Findings

The MR angiogram demonstrates the presence of left internal carotid artery stenosis of an unusual morphology, best seen on the select rotation views (Figs. 6A–C). The complex nature of the lesion included the orifice of the external carotid artery as well.

Diagnosis

Complex stenotic lesion of left common carotid bifurcation.

Discussion

The exact morphology of carotid lesions may be difficult to ascertain with MR angiography alone. In this particular case, a complex lesion was demonstrated with significant stenosis. However, the areas of ulceration (*arrows*) were difficult to detect until the intraarterial angiogram was performed (Fig. 6D). This points out the fact that MR angiography provides information on the basis of both anatomic and physiologic data. The turbulence-induced dephasing of spins may preclude definitive evaluation of lesion morphology with MR angiographic sequences. Thus, for purposes of preoperative planning, intraarterial angiography may still be necessary. Certainly, if the patient remains symptomatic in the face of a negative MR angiogram, an intraarterial angiogram should also be done to detect subtle pathology such as minor ulcerations or fibromuscular disease.

References

1. Masaryk AM, Ross JS, et al. 3DFT MR angiography of the carotid bifurcation: potential and limitations as a screening examination. *Radiology* 1991;179:797–804.
2. Anderson CM, Saloner D, et al. Assessment of carotid artery stenosis by MR angiography: comparison with x-ray angiography and color-coded Doppler ultrasound. *AJNR* 1992;13:989–1003.
3. Heiserman JE, Drayer BP, et al. Carotid artery stenosis: clinical efficacy of two-dimensional time-of-flight MR angiography. *Radiology* 1992;182:761–768.

Submitted by: Michael Brant-Zawadzki, M.D., F.A.C.R., Hoag Memorial Hospital, Newport Beach, California; Michael Brant-Zawadzki, M.D., F.A.C.R., Senior Editor.

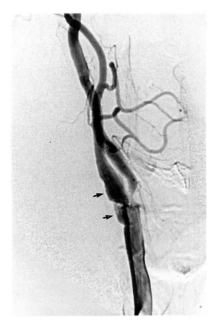

FIG. 6D. Intraarterial DSA LCA injection.

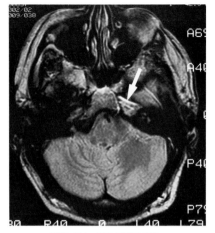

FIG. 7A. SE 2900/30.

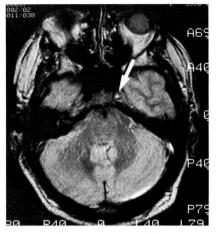

FIG. 7B. SE 2900/30.

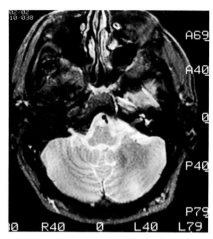

FIG. 7C. SE 2900/80.

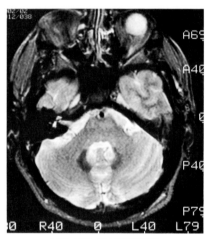

FIG. 7D. SE 2900/80.

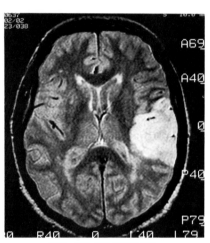

FIG. 7E. SE 2900/30.

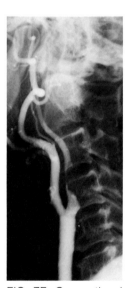

FIG. 7F. Conventional angiogram (left ICA).

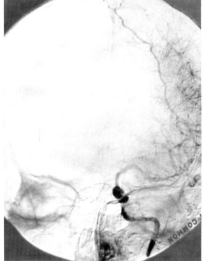

FIG. 7G. Conventional angiogram (LICA).

Clinical History

A 64-year-old male with expressive aphasia.

Findings

Intermediate weighted images show intraluminal hyperintense signal in the left internal carotid artery (ICA) (Figs. 7A and B, *arrows*). On T2-weighted images there is persisting signal in the horizontal portion of the left ICA (Fig. 7C) and a partial central flow void with peripheral rim of hyperintense signal (Fig. 7D). The caliber of the left ICA is decreased compared to the right. Axial intermediate weighted image (Fig. 7E) shows a wedge-shaped lesion in the distribution of the left middle cerebral artery (MCA). Flow void is present in the MCA branches.

Left common carotid (CC) angiogram shows a greater than 95% stenosis with decreased caliber of the distal cervical ICA. The intracranial portion of the left ICA (Fig. 7F) shows washout, as does the MCA proximal to the trifurction (Fig. 7G).

Diagnosis

Acute left MCA infarct with high-grade left cervical ICA stenosis.

Discussion

The presence of intracranial arterial flow void is a normal finding (1), but an extracranial cervical carotid arterial lesion can still be present (2). A partial flow void in the petrous or cavernous portion of the intracranial ICA can be associated with extracranial cervical ICA disease as illustrated by this case.

The peripheral increased signal in a vessel has been reported to represent a "boundary layer signal" of peripheral more slowly moving protons and the central hypointensity as being representative of higher velocity protons (3). It must be appreciated that with a high-grade cervical ICA stenosis there is overall slower flow downstream, thus not only affecting the signal behavior of the normally expected intracranial arterial flow void but also the vessel caliber size. On conventional angiography this reduction in flow can be appreciated as earlier contrast flow into the external carotid artery branches overlaying the calvarium compared to intracranial ICA branches.

The peripheral hyperintensity of the partial flow void is not felt to represent thrombus (3). A decrease in vessel caliber should be looked for on all MR images as indicative of decreased flow. The presence of signal intensity in the entire ICA (loss of entire flow void) suggests complete occlusion (3), but can also represent severe but not near-total occlusion (2), as this case illustrates with the signal in the horizontal portion of the left ICA.

References

1. Bradley WG Jr. Flow phenomena in MR imaging. *AJR* 1988;150:983–994.
2. Brant-Zawadzki M. Routine MR imaging of the internal carotid siphon: angiographic correlation with cervical carotid lesions. *AJNR* 1990;11:467–471.
3. Heinz ER, Yeates AE, Djang WT. Significant extracranial carotid stenosis: detection on routine cerebral MR images. *Radiology* 1989;170:843–848.

Submitted by: Orest B. Boyko, M.D., Ph.D., Duke University Medical Center, Durham, North Carolina; Michael Brant-Zawadzki, M.D., F.A.C.R., Senior Editor.

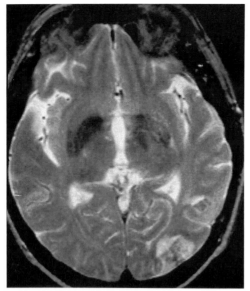

FIG. 8A. Axial SE 2500/90.

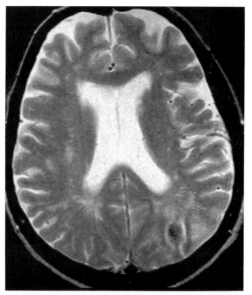

FIG. 8B. Axial SE 2500/90.

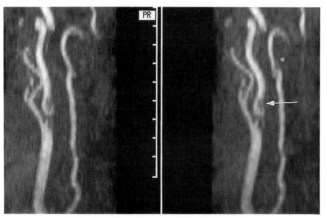

FIG. 8C. 2D TOF (FLASH) 38/9/30°.

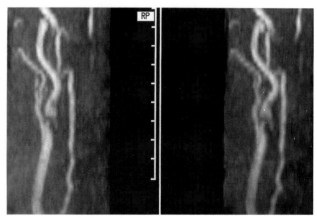

FIG. 8D. 2D TOF (FLASH) 38/9/30°.

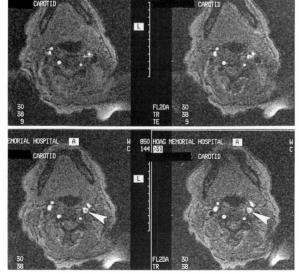

FIG. 8E. 2D TOF (FLASH) 38/9/30°.

Clinical History

A 67-year-old female with left middle cerebral artery infarction.

Findings

Selected T2-weighted axial (second echo) images (Figs. 8A and B) demonstrate left posterior temporal ischemic changes with low signal intensity in the superior slice (Fig. 8B) within the watershed region of the posterior and middle cerebral artery distribution.

The accompanying MR angiographic study of the left internal carotid artery (Fig. 8C) shows a stenosis as well as findings suggestive of a filling defect (*arrow*) just above the stenotic segment. Notice that some of the rotations accentuate the area of stenosis (Fig. 8D).

The individual partitions (Fig. 8E) strongly suggest an intraluminal defect in the left internal carotid artery (*arrowheads*).

Diagnosis

Severe atherosclerotic plaque with intraluminal component and associated stenosis.

Discussion

At surgery, a severe stenosis was found with a large atherosclerotic plaque encroaching on the lumen of the left internal carotid artery. Note that both the MR and intraarterial angiogram (Fig. 8F) are highly suggestive of an intraluminal clot. The plaque was found to be ladened with cholesterol, possibly explaining the embolic infarction of the brain.

Incidentally, this patient returned several months after surgery with complete occlusion of the left common carotid artery as demonstrated on the follow-up MR angiogram (Fig. 8G).

References

1. Heiserman LE, Drayer BP, et al. Carotid artery stenosis: clinical efficacy of two-dimensional time-of-flight MR angiography. *Radiology* 1992;182:761–768.
2. Anderson CM, Saloner D, et al. Assessment of carotid artery stenosis by MR angiography: comparison with x-ray angiography and color coded Doppler ultrasound. *AJNR* 1992;13:984–1003.
3. Litt AW, Eidelman EM, et al. Diagnosis of carotid artery stenosis: comparison of 2DFT time-of-flight MR angiography with contrast angiography in 50 patients. *AJNR* 1991;12:149–154.

Submitted by: Michael Brant-Zawadzki, M.D., F.A.C.R., Hoag Memorial Hospital, Newport Beach, California; Michael Brant-Zawadzki, M.D., F.A.C.R., Senior Editor.

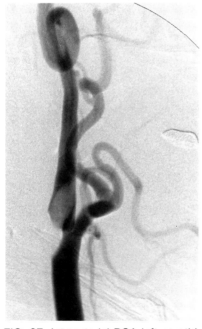

FIG. 8F. Intraarterial DSA left carotid art. injection.

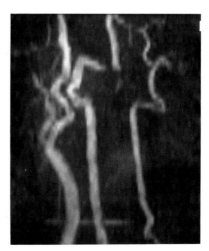

FIG. 8G. 2D TOF (FLASH) 38/9/30.

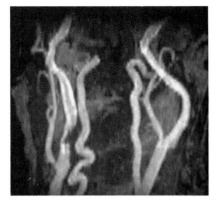

FIG. 9A. 3D TOF (FISP) 43/8/20°.

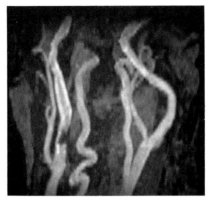

FIG. 9B. 3D TOF (FISP) 43/8/20°.

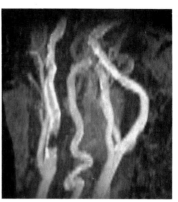

FIG. 9C. 3D TOF (FISP) 43/8/20°.

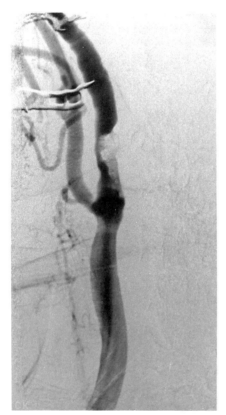

FIG. 9D. Intraarterial DSA-RCA injection.

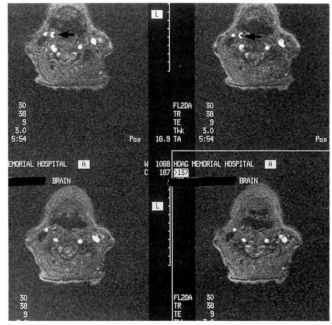

FIG. 9E. 3D TOF (FISP) 43/8/20°.

Clinical History

An 84-year-old female with left- and right-sided amaurosis fugax and transient left-sided weakness.

Findings

The 2D time-of-flight magnetic resonance angiogram (MRA) of the neck utilizing magnetization transfer suppression and variable flip angle technique (512 matrix) nicely demonstrates a severe focal stenosis of the right internal carotid artery on the three rotations selected (Figs. 9A–C). Indeed, the lesion appears possibly intraluminal.

The intraarterial angiogram (Fig. 9D) performed 2 days later also suggests an intraluminal filling defect in this severely diseased vessel. The individual partitions from the MRA study demonstrate the lesion as a progressive obliteration of the right internal carotid artery trunk, but the obliteration appears extrinsic (Fig. 9E, *arrow*).

Diagnosis

Severe atherosclerotic plaque producing preocclusive stenosis, simulating intraluminal thrombus.

Discussion

This case points out the value of the cross-sectional partition images from the MRA study in helping characterize a lesion as intra- versus extraluminal. This differentiation can be difficult with MR and even intraarterial angiography (see Case 16).

Incidentally, the choice of 3D technique with a 512 matrix helps diminish the pixel size and thus minimize intravoxel dephasing. This more accurately depicts the degree of stenosis as opposed to the conventional 2D time-of-flight techniques, which exaggerate such stenosis on the basis of dephasing (Fig. 9F).

References

1. Masaryk TJ, Modic MT, et al. Three-dimensional (volume) gradient-echo imaging of the carotid bifurcation: preliminary clinical experience. *Radiology* 1989;171:801–806.
2. Lett AW, Edelman EM, et al. Diagnosis of carotid artery stenosis: comparison of 2DFT time-of-flight MR angiography with contrast angiography in 50 patients. *AJR* 1991;156:611–616.
3. Edelman R, Mattle HP, et al. MR angiography. *AJR* 1990;154:937–946.

Submitted by: Michael Brant-Zawadzki, M.D., F.A.C.R., Hoag Memorial Hospital, Newport Beach, California; Michael Brant-Zawadzki, M.D., F.A.C.R., Senior Editor.

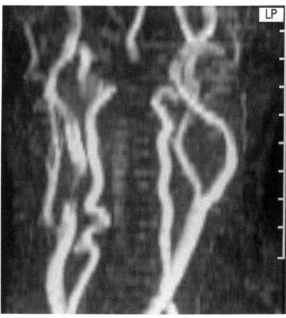

FIG. 9F. 20 TOF (FLASH) 38/9/30°.

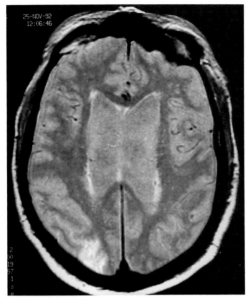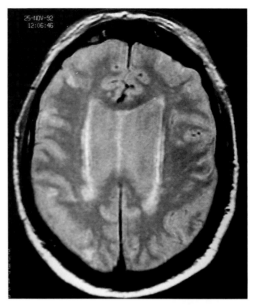

FIG. 10A. Axial turbo SE 3500/19.　　　　FIG. 10B. Axial turbo SE 3500/19.

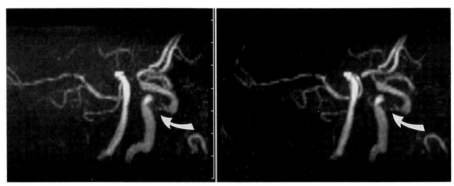

FIG. 10C. 3D TOF 43/8/20° MTS, TONE-two rotations.

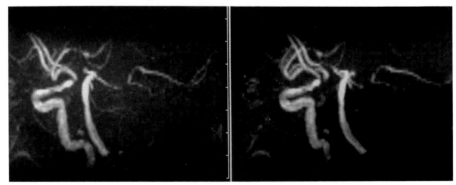

FIG. 10D. 3D TOF 43/8/20° MTS, TONE-two rotations.

Clinical History

A 76-year-old male with recent right hemispheric cerebrovascular accident (CVA).

Findings

The axial T2-weighted spin-echo images (first echo) show evidence of signal alteration in the posterior right temporal-occipital region consistent with a recent ischemic event (Figs. 10A and B). The MR angiogram showed no significant pathology in the neck, but did demonstrate a focal area of flow alteration and void in the carotid siphon of the right internal carotid segment (Fig. 10C, *arrows*). In contradistinction, the left side showed no such defect (Fig. 10D).

Diagnosis

Severe atheromatous stenosis of right internal carotid cavernous segment.

Discussion

This case documents the importance of evaluating the cervicocranial vessels in their full extent, rather than in just the neck (such as with Doppler ultrasound). In this case, the cavernous segment lesion was responsible for the infarct. The cavernous segment of the ICA is prone to artifact due to dephasing from turbulent flow and magnetic susceptibility effects. An intraarterial angiogram was performed (Fig. 10E), which confirmed the MRA findings.

Incidentally, transorbital Doppler did verify the presence of accelerated velocities in the clinoid carotid artery.

References

1. Polak JF, Bajakian RL, et al. Detection of internal carotid artery stenosis: comparison of MR angiography, color Doppler sonography and arteriography. *Radiology* 1992;182:35–40.
2. Anderson CM, Saloner I, et al. Assessment of carotid artery stenosis by MR angiography and color-coded Doppler ultrasound. *AJNR* 1992;13:989–1003.
3. Brant-Zawadzki MN, Gillan G. Extracranial carotid magnetic resonance angiography. *Cardiovasc Intervent Radiol* 1991;15:82–90.

Submitted by: Michael Brant-Zawadzki, M.D., F.A.C.R., Hoag Memorial Hospital, Newport Beach, California; Michael Brant-Zawadzki, M.D., F.A.C.R., Senior Editor.

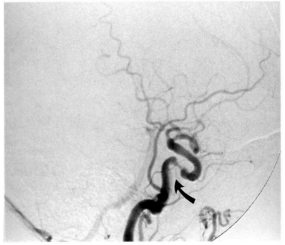

FIG. 10E. Intraarterial angiogram right carotid artery injection.

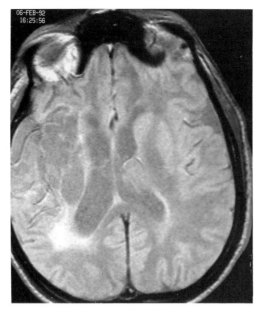

FIG. 11A. Axial SE 2500/22.

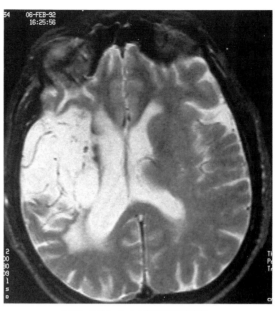

FIG. 11B. Axial SE 2500/90.

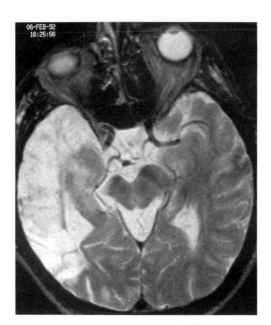

FIG. 11C. Axial SE 2500/90.

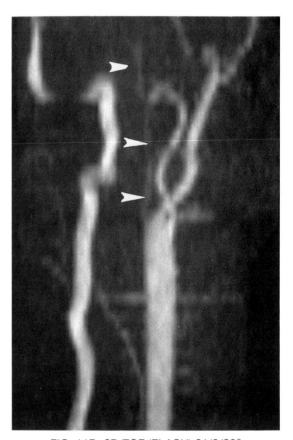

FIG. 11D. 2D TOF (FLASH) 31/9/30°.

Clinical History

A 57-year-old with prior middle right cerebral artery infarction, now presents with recurrent transient ischemic attacks (TIAs).

Findings

Selected T2-weighted first and second echo images (Figs. 11A and B) demonstrate cystic encephalomalacia in the distribution of the right middle cerebral artery system. Note that there are middle cerebral artery branches present through the area of infarction, as evidenced by serpentine channels with signal void. In addition, patency of the right supraclinoid carotid artery is demonstrated on the adjacent lower image (Fig. 11C). The 2D time-of-flight angiography with traveling saturation pulse shows what appears to be complete occlusion of the right carotid (Fig. 11D). However, a very thin "string" is suggested in the region of the expected internal carotid artery branch (*arrowheads*).

Diagnosis

Complete right internal carotid artery occlusion with simulation of the "string sign."

Discussion

The intraarterial angiogram (Fig. 11E), done because of the difficulty in excluding a very thin remnant right internal carotid artery, demonstrates that the "string" is actually due to the ascending pharyngeal branch (*arrowheads*) of the right external carotid artery. Left vertebral artery intraarterial angiogram shows that the patency of the supraclinoid carotid artery is explainable on the basis of collateral flow through the posterior communicating artery from the vertebral basilar system. Note good filling of the middle cerebral artery (Fig. 11F) and its branches via this route, explaining the serpentine vessel patency seen on the conventional MRI study.

This study again demonstrates some difficulty in absolute certainty regarding complete occlusion versus some residual patency for the internal carotid artery system on the basis of MR angiography alone. In cases where symptoms warrant, intraarterial angiography may still need to be done to completely evaluate the circulation to the brain.

References

1. Heiserman JE, Drayer BP, et al. Carotid artery stenosis: clinical efficacy of two-dimensional time-of-flight MR angiography. *Radiology* 1992;182:761–768.
2. Lett AW, Edelman EM, et al. Diagnosis of carotid artery stenosis: comparison of 2DFT time-of-flight MR angiography with contrast angiography in 50 patients. *AJNR* 1991;12:149–154.
3. Masaryk TJ, Modic MT, et al. Three-dimensional (volume) gradient-echo imaging of the carotid bifurcation: preliminary clinical experience. *Radiology* 1989;171:801–806.

Submitted by: Michael Brant-Zawadzki, M.D., F.A.C.R., Hoag Memorial Hospital, Newport Beach, California; Michael Brant-Zawadzki, M.D., F.A.C.R., Senior Editor.

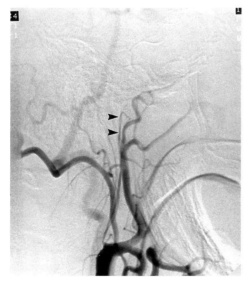

FIG. 11E. Intraarterial DSA RCA.

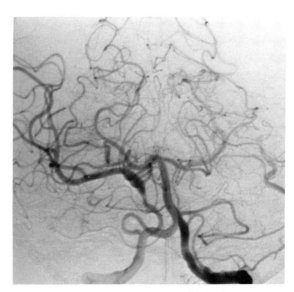

FIG. 11F. Intraarterial DSA LVA.

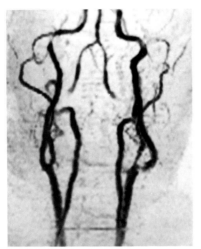

FIG. 12A. 2D TOF MRA, 45/9.

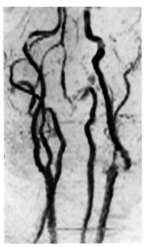

FIG. 12B. 2D TOF MRA, 45/9.

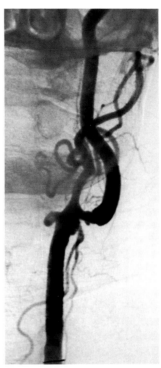

FIG. 12C. Left CCA angiogram.

Clinical History

A 71-year-old female with history of transient ischemic attacks (TIAs).

Findings

The 2D time-of-flight (TOF) magnetic resonance angiography (MRA) reveals on 3D stacked images apparent lack of flow in a segment of the proximal left internal carotid artery (ICA) at the carotid bifurcation, suggesting high-grade stenosis (Figs. 12A and B). The presence of distal flow-related enhancement (FRE) in the left ICA excludes a complete occlusion.

Conventional left common carotid angiogram (CCA) in the anterior posterior (AP) projection reveals only a 60% stenosis with focal ulceration (Fig. 12C).

Diagnosis

Moderate atherosclerotic luminal narrowing of the left ICA with focal ulceration.

Discussion

This case illustrates the tendency of 2D TOF MRA to "overestimate" a stenosis by signal loss from intravoxel dephasing at the level of atherosclerotic change. In addition the 2D TOF MRA partition images were acquired axially and the anatomical course of the proximal left ICA is nearly horizontal and thus parallel with the axial slice. This can lead to signal loss due to saturation effects of in-plane flow.

References

1. Keller PJ, Drayer BP, Fram EK, et al. MR angiography with two-dimensional acquisition and three-dimensional display—work in progress. *Radiology* 1989;173:527–532.
2. Anderson CM, Saloner D, Tsuruda JS, et al. Artifacts in maximum-intensity-projection display of MR angiograms. *AJR* 1990;154:623–629.

Submitted by: Orest B. Boyko, M.D., Ph.D., Duke University Medical Center, Durham, North Carolina; Michael Brant-Zawadzki, M.D., F.A.C.R., Senior Editor.

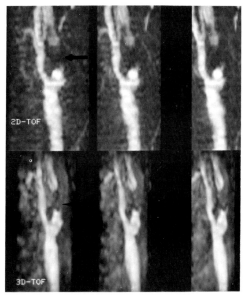

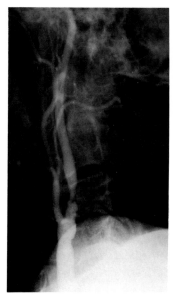

FIG. 13A. 2D TOF MRA (top) and 3D TOF MRA (bottom), 3-D reprojections.

FIG. 13B. Conventional angiogram, L CCA.

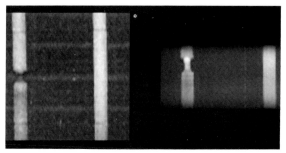

FIG. 13C. Flow phantom with stenotic segment in right channel studied by 2D TOF (Left) and 3D TOF (Right) MRA.

Clinical History

A 64-year-old male with transient ischemic attacks (TIAs).

Findings

Magnetic resonance angiography (MRA) using 2D time-of-flight (TOF) (Fig. 13A *top, arrow*) and 3D TOF MRA (Fig. 13A *bottom, arrowhead*) both show discontinuity of the flow-related enhancement in left internal carotid artery (ICA). Conventional angiogram reveals ulcerated plaque (Fig. 13B) and greater than 90% stenosis (Fig. 13B) of the left ICA.

Diagnosis

Atherosclerosis with severe stenosis and ulcerated atherosclerotic plaque of the left ICA.

Discussion

The 2D TOF and 3D TOF MRA (1,2) provide useful images of carotid arteries in the neck and both imaging techniques utilize gradient recalled echo pulse sequences that suppress stationary proton signal but are very sensitive to flowing spins into the imaging plane (flow-related enhancement). Note the lack of visualization of bony anatomy on MRA, which is readily identifiable on the conventional angiogram. Also, note the better depiction of irregularity and ulceration in the proximal internal carotid artery on the conventional angiogram. Both 2D and 3D TOF MRA techniques are susceptible to lack of visualization of the actual stenotic segment on postprocessed maximum-intensity-projection (MIP) images (Fig. 13A) partly related to signal loss due to intravoxel dephasing. This has been described for both 2D TOF and 3D TOF (3). Although the actual stenosis cannot be seen, the suggestion can be made of a stenosis of at least greater than 70%. Because the voxels are larger with typical 2D TOF MRA than with 3D TOF MRA, greater intravoxel dephasing occurs on 2D TOF images. This can exaggerate stenosis due to signal loss, as shown on the phantom (Fig. 13C). The 2D TOF MRA of the stenotic flow phantom segment greatly overestimates the lesion shown by the 3D TOF MRA study.

References

1. Keller PJ, Drayer BP, Fram EK, et al. MR angiography with two-dimensional acquisition and three-dimensional display: work in progress. *Radiology* 1989;173:527–532.
2. Schmalbrock P, Yuan C, Chakeres DW, et al. Volume MR angiography: methods to achieve very short echo times. *Radiology* 1990;175:861–865.
3. Boyko OB, Edelman RR, Litt AW. MR angiography of the carotid arteries: clinical applications. *RSNA Today Video* 1991;5(2).

Submitted by: Orest B. Boyko, M.D., Ph.D., Duke University Medical Center, Durham, North Carolina; Michael Brant-Zawadzki, M.D., F.A.C.R., Senior Editor.

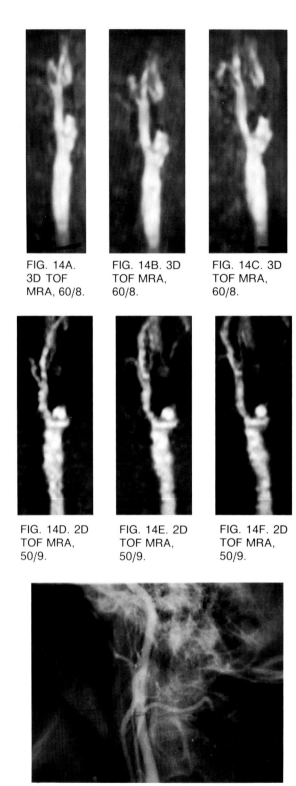

FIG. 14A. 3D TOF MRA, 60/8.

FIG. 14B. 3D TOF MRA, 60/8.

FIG. 14C. 3D TOF MRA, 60/8.

FIG. 14D. 2D TOF MRA, 50/9.

FIG. 14E. 2D TOF MRA, 50/9.

FIG. 14F. 2D TOF MRA, 50/9.

FIG. 14G. Conventional left CCA.

Clinical History

A 64-year-old male with transient ischemic attacks (TIAs) (same patient as in Case 13).

Findings

The 3D time-of-flight (TOF) magnetic resonance angiography (MRA) 3D reprojection images show discontinuity of flow in the proximal left internal carotid artery (ICA) but with distal flow-related enhancement (FRE) showing patency of the distal ICA (Figs. 14A–C). Similar findings are present on the 2D TOF MRA 3D reprojections (Figs. 14D–F). Conventional left common carotid angiogram (CCA) shows a greater atherosclerotic plaque with possible ulceration and greater than 90% stenosis (Fig. 14G).

Diagnosis

Left internal carotid origin stenosis and ulceration.

Discussion

The clinical utility of 3D TOF (1) and 2D TOF (2) MRA in imaging the carotid artery bifurcation is currently undergoing evaluation. Both techniques are susceptible to signal loss due to intravoxel dephasing, which is accentuated by velocity variation due to higher order motion (acceleration turbulence) which occurs in the region of vascular stenoses (see Case B). Atherosclerotic plaque ulceration can be best detected in patients using conventional angiography, although it can miss ulceration in up to 30% of patients (3). It is unlikely that either 2D or 3D TOF will be more sensitive for detecting ulceration.

References

1. Masaryk AM, Ross JS, DiCello MC, et al. 3DFT MR angiography of the carotid bifurcation: potential and limitations as a screening examination. *Radiology* 1991;179:797–804.
2. Litt AW, Eidelman EM, Pinto RS, et al. Diagnosis of carotid artery stenosis: comparison of 2DFT time-of-flight MR angiography with contrast angiography in 50 patients. *AJNR* 1991;12:149–154.
3. Eikelboom BC, Riles TR, Mintzer R, et al. Inaccuracy of angiography in the diagnosis of carotid ulceration. *Stroke* 1983;14:882–885.

Submitted by: Orest B. Boyko, M.D., Ph.D., Duke University Medical Center, Durham, North Carolina; Michael Brant-Zawadzki, M.D., F.A.C.R., Senior Editor.

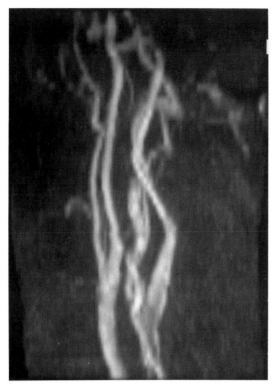

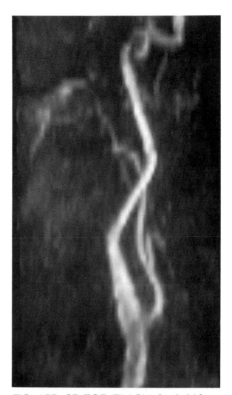

FIG. 15A. 2D TOF (FLASH) 31/9/30° RPO rotation.

FIG. 15B. 2D TOF (FLASH) 31/9/30°.

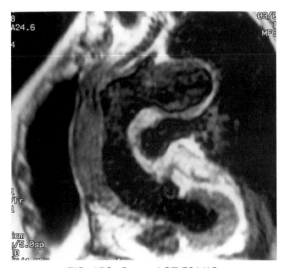

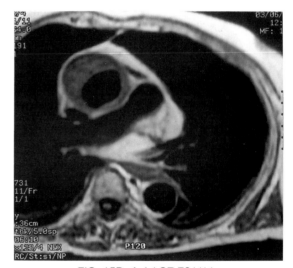

FIG. 15C. Coronal SE 731/12.

FIG. 15D. Axial SE 731/11.

Clinical History

A 77-year-old female with a history of hypertension now presenting with sudden left hemiparesis and loss of consciousness.

Findings

An MR angiogram (Fig. 15A) in the right posterior oblique rotation demonstrates what appears to be a filling defect in the distal right common carotid artery which branches into the bifurcation. This is better shown on the select view (Fig. 15B).

Due to mediastinal widening on the chest x-ray, a conventional thoracic MR study was done, which demonstrates a chronic dissection involving the ascending aorta (Figs. 15C and D).

Diagnosis

Embolic filling defect, right common carotid artery.

Discussion

Twenty-five percent of all aortic dissections present with neurological symptoms. In this particular case, the cause was an embolic event from the aortic dissection. An intraarterial angiogram was performed, which demonstrates partial occlusion of the right subclavian artery as well (Fig. 15E). The patient's inability to cooperate precluded definitive study of the right carotid artery.

Reference

1. Kadir S. Arteriography of the thoracic aorta. In: *Diagnostic angiography.* Philadelphia: WB Saunders, 1986; 124–171.

Submitted by: Michael Brant-Zawadzki, M.D., F.A.C.R., Hoag Memorial Hospital, Newport Beach, California; Michael Brant-Zawadzki, M.D., F.A.C.R., Senior Editor.

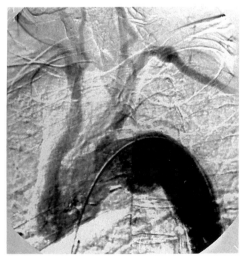

FIG. 15E. Intraarterial DSA aortic arch injection.

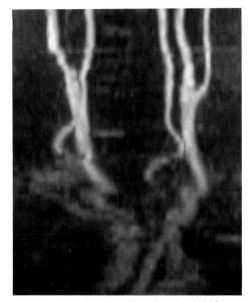

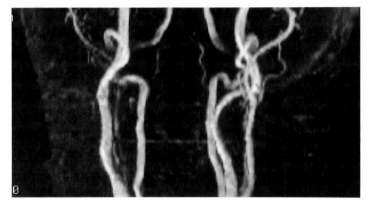

FIG. 16A. 2D TOF (FLASH) 31/9/30°.

FIG. 16B. 2D TOF (GRASS) 45°/9/60°.

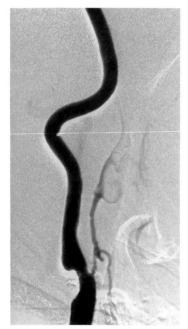

FIG. 16C. Intraarterial DSA RCA injection.

Clinical History

A 72-year-old female with right hemispheric transient ischemic attacks (TIAs) and suspected preocclusive lesion on carotid ultrasound examination.

Findings

The MR angiogram (Fig. 16A) demonstrates unremarkable appearance of the left common carotid artery and its bifurcation. The right common carotid artery bifurcation shows what appears to be a "string sign" of the internal carotid artery. However, on closer inspection this "string sign" actually represents the external carotid as opposed to the internal carotid artery. The internal carotid artery shows a normal-appearing lumen, which is irregular at its origin. A second acquisition was obtained (Fig. 16B) with higher centering, which verifies this impression.

Diagnosis

Right external carotid artery occlusion.

Discussion

Ultrasound may have difficulty differentiating internal and external carotid artery on the basis of anatomic or flow-velocity data. MR imaging has the advantage of seeing a longer portion of the vessel anatomy and better orienting the vessel in question to the rest of the neck and brain. In this case, the original MR acquisition was somewhat low for optimal delineation of the distal carotid anatomy. The higher acquisition verified the impression of external carotid artery as opposed to internal carotid artery stenosis, which was verified with intraarterial angiography (Fig. 16C).

References

1. Anderson CM, Saloner D, et al. Assessment of carotid artery stenosis by MR angiography: comparison with x-ray angiography and color-coded Doppler ultrasound. *AJNR* 1992;13:989–1003.
2. Litt AW, Edelman EM, et al. Diagnosis of carotid artery stenosis: comparison of 2DFT time-of-flight MR angiography with contrast angiography in 50 patients. *AJNR* 1991;12:149–154.
3. Heiserman JE, Drayer BP, et al. Carotid artery stenosis: clinical efficacy of two-dimensional time-of-flight MR angiography. *Radiology* 1992;182:761–768.

Submitted by: Michael Brant-Zawadzki, M.D., F.A.C.R., Hoag Memorial Hospital, Newport Beach, California; Michael Brant-Zawadzki, M.D., F.A.C.R., Senior Editor.

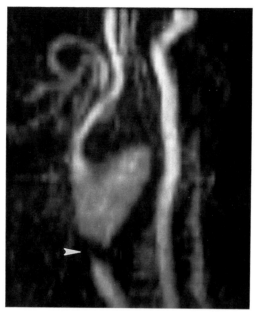

FIG. 17A. 20 TDF (FLASH) 36/10/30°.

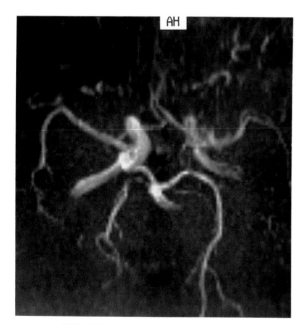

FIG. 17B. 30 TOF (FISP) 40/7/15°.

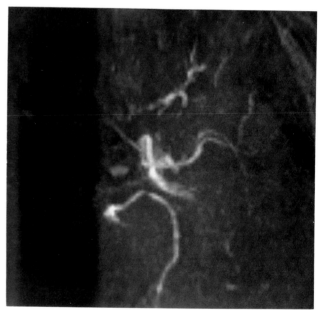

FIG. 17C. 3D TOF (FISP) 40/7/15°.

Clinical History

A 69-year-old male status post–left carotid endarterectomy with recent transient ischemic attack (TIA), and nondefinitive carotid ultrasound.

Findings

The selected, postprocessed image (maximum intensity pixel algorithm) view of the left side of the neck (Fig. 17A) shows the distal common carotid with a focal flow void defect (*arrowhead*), completely obliterating the vessel lumen, just at the base of a large outpouching at the expected location of the endarterectomy and distal internal carotid artery. There is no visualization of distal internal carotid artery flow. The adjacent left vertebral artery is unremarkable. The intracranial 3D time-of-flight study (Fig. 17B) demonstrates flow in both the right and the left middle cerebral artery and carotid artery siphons. Utilization of selective presaturation of the right carotid circulation (Fig. 17C), shows that flow is present in the left carotid artery and its branches to the brain; this indicates collateralization by at least the basilar route visualized on this study.

The intraarterial angiographic study (Fig. 17D) verified the pseudoaneurysm at the surgical site. Note that there is a narrow channel just at the base of the pseudoaneurysm (*arrow*), where the magnetic resonance angiogram (MRA) shows a complete lack of flow. This overestimation of narrowing on the MRA is caused by a combination of turbulent flow through the stenotic segment, and the presence of surgical clips with alteration of magnetic field homogeneity at this site. The intracranial view (Fig. 17E) demonstrates collateralization of the carotid artery through the ophthalmic route (*arrow*) (in addition to the basilar route demonstrated on MRA), explaining the reconstitution of a long segment of the precavernous and cavernous left carotid artery.

Diagnosis

Postsurgical pseudoaneurysm at site of carotid endarterectomy, with complete internal carotid artery occlusion. Reconstitution of intracranial flow through external carotid and posterior fossa circulations.

Discussion

The large pseudoaneurysm at the site of surgery precluded a definitive ultrasound evaluation, as the highly unusual flow pattern through this region was confusing. The MRA solved the issues; however, it did overestimate the degree of stenosis at the base of the pseudoaneurysm for reasons mentioned above. Note that when the carotid siphon is reconstituted to the petrous portion, the possibility of a "string sign" should be raised (collapsed cervical internal carotid artery rather than occluded vessel). Therefore, one must be certain that no patent lumen is available for surgical correction. This can occasionally be verified with MRA but whenever a question arises, intraarterial angiography still needs to be done for complete assurance that no potential for surgical reperfusion is available.

The use of saturation pulses is one method that allows evaluation of the dynamics of flow on MRA examinations. Note, however, that the ophthalmic collateralization of the internal carotid artery is quite difficult to ascertain with routine MRA sequences. Specific sequences for evaluation of flow direction include phase contrast techniques.

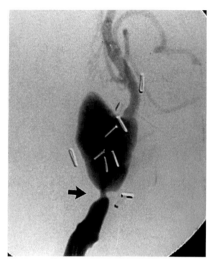

FIG. 17D. Conventional DSA LCA.

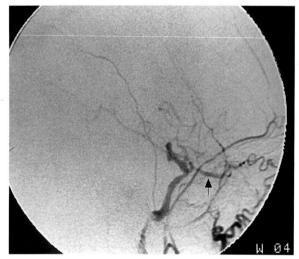

FIG. 17E. Conventional DSA LCA.

References

1. Edelman RR, Mattle HP, et al. MR angiography. *AJR* 1990;154:937–946.
2. Anderson CM, Saloner D, et al. Artifacts of maximum intensity projection display of MR angiograms. *AJR* 1990;154:623–629.
3. Edelman RR, Wentz KU, et al. Intracerebral anteriovenous malformations: evaluation with selective MR angiography and venography. *Radiology* 1989;173:831–837.
4. Felmlee JP, Ehman RL. Spatial presaturation: a method for suppressing flow artifacts and improving depiction of vascular anatomy in MR imaging. *Radiology* 1987;164:559–564.

Submitted by: Michael Brant-Zawadzki, M.D., F.A.C.R., Hoag Memorial Hospital, Newport Beach, California; Michael Brant-Zawadzki, M.D., F.A.C.R., Senior Editor.

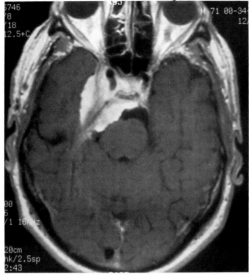
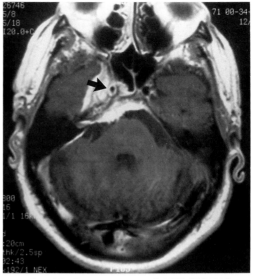

FIG. 18A. Postcontrast axial SE 800/16.   FIG. 18B. Postcontrast axial SE 800/116.

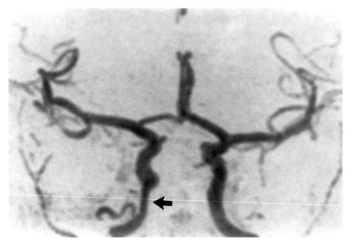
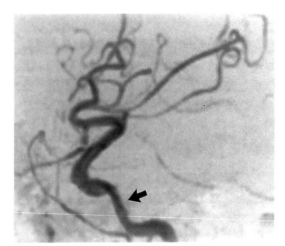

FIG. 18C. 3D TOF MOTSA 31/5.3/30°.   FIG. 18D. 3D TOF MOTSA 31/5.3/30°.

Clinical History

A 71-year-old male with decreasing vision in the right eye, and a right sixth nerve palsy.

Findings

Enhancing lesion with irregular margins is seen involving the right cavernous sinus (Fig. 18A). The lower sections demonstrate apparent narrowing of the precavernous right internal carotid artery (Fig. 18B, *arrow*). The 3D multiple overlapping thin slab acquisition (MOTSA) angiography verifies the narrowing of the right precavernous carotid artery segment (Figs. 18C and D, *arrow*). An intraarterial angiogram verifies the narrowed precavernous carotid artery segment and also shows subtle blush surrounding it (Fig. 18E).

Diagnosis

Right cavernous dural meningioma, with right internal carotid artery encasement.

Discussion

This is a typical appearance for a cavernous dural meningioma with homogeneous enhancement and involvement of the paracavernous region, including the extension into the middle fossa and the prepontine space. Meningiomas in this location will typically narrow the carotid artery by encasement, a strong differentiating feature when compared to other lesions such as pituitary adenomas. The classic blush seen on the intraarterial angiogram and demonstration of the feeding vessels (in this case small cavernous segment branches from the internal carotid artery) helps in determining the diagnosis.

References

1. Yeakley JW, Kulkarni MV, et al. High-resolution MR imaging of juxtasellar meningiomas with CT and angiographic correlation. *AJNR* 1988;9:279–285.
2. Young SC, Grossman RI, et al. MR of vascular encasement in parasellar masses: comparison with angiography and CT. *AJNR* 1988;9:35–38.
3. Bradac GB, Riva A, et al. Cavernous sinus meningiomas: an MRI study. *Neuroradiology* 1987;29:578–581.

Submitted by: Evan Framm, M.D., Barrows Neurological Institute, St. Joseph's Hospital, Phoenix, Arizona; Michael Brant-Zawadzki, M.D., F.A.C.R., Senior Editor.

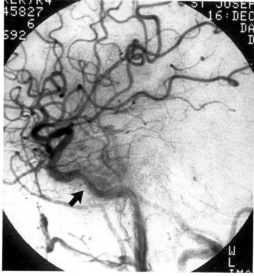

FIG. 18E. Intraarterial DSA RCA injection.

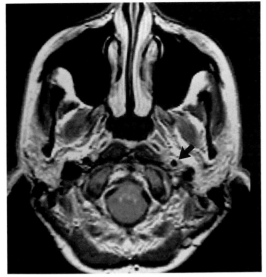

FIG. 19A. Axial SE 2800/22.

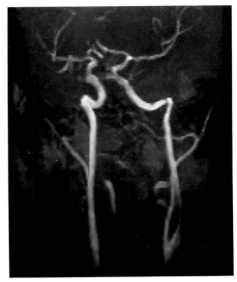

FIG. 19B. Coronal 3D TOF (FISP) 30/7/15°.

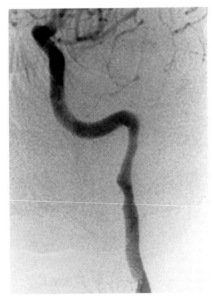

FIG. 19C. Intraarterial DSA angiogram LCA.

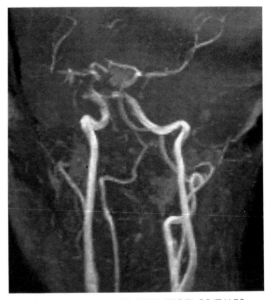

FIG. 19D. Coronal 3D TOF (FISP) 30/7/15°.

Clinical History

A 32-year-old female with sudden onset of left-sided Horner's syndrome and blurred vision.

Findings

The first echo image (Fig. 19A) of the T2-weighted sequence at the level of the skull base is normal. Specifically, note the normal appearance of the signal void in the immediate subcranial portion of the internal carotid arteries. There is a suggestion of slight diminution of the left internal carotid artery lumen (*arrow*) when compared to the right, but this can only be equivocally discerned in retrospect.

The magnetic resonance angiographic (MRA) (Fig. 19B) study demonstrates fusiform narrowing of the subtemporal portion of the left internal carotid artery system compared to the normal-appearing right side. The subsequent intraarterial angiogram (Fig. 19C) verifies the presence of localized narrowing and irregularity of this portion of the carotid artery. The follow-up MRA study (Fig. 19D) obtained 4 months later demonstrates resolution of the narrowing.

Diagnosis

Carotid dissection.

Discussion

A high index of suspicion was necessary to proceed with the MR angiographic study in this case, as the classic narrowing of the internal carotid artery with intramural hematoma is not present on the conventional spin-echo sequences. Nevertheless, given the history, MR angiography was done and verified the presence of findings consistent with dissection. An intraarterial angiogram was also performed, as this was early in the experience with MRA. The follow-up MRA study documents the typical resolution of dissection. The patient was treated with anticoagulants during this period. Her symptoms completely resolved.

Carotid dissection typically occurs high in the cervical portion of the vessel, where it is "tethered" by the bony canal of the temporal calvarium. One must be careful in interpreting the petrous portion of the carotid arteries, as artifactual signal dropout and narrowing can occur in this segment due to magnetic susceptibility effects and turbulence within the tortuous segment of the vessel (see Case 27).

References

1. Quisling RG, Friedman WA, Rhoton AL Jr. High cervical carotid artery dissection: spontaneous resolution. *AJNR* 1980;1:463–468.
2. Wagle WA, Dumoulin CL, et al. 3DFT MR angiography of carotid and basilar arteries. *AJNR* 1989;10:911–919.
3. Brant-Zawadzki MN, Gillan G. Extracranial carotid magnetic resonance angiography. *Cardiovasc Intervent Radiol* 1992;15:82–90.
4. Nguyen Bui L, Brant-Zawadzki M. MR angiography of cervico-cranial dissection. *Stroke* 1993;24:126–131.

Submitted by: Michael Brant-Zawadzki, M.D., F.A.C.R., Hoag Memorial Hospital, Newport Beach, California; Michael Brant-Zawadzki, M.D., F.A.C.R., Senior Editor.

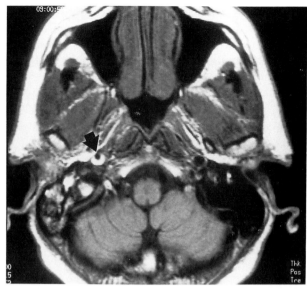

FIG. 20A. Axial SE 700/15.

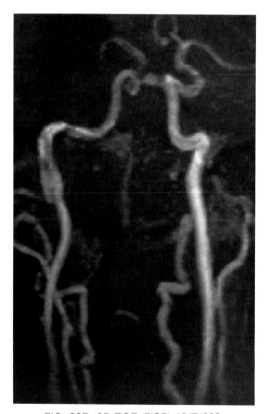

FIG. 20B. 3D TOF (FISP) 40/7/30°.

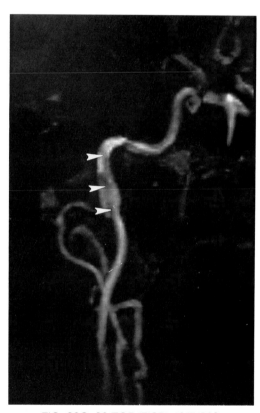

FIG. 20C. 30 TOF (FISP) 40/7/30°.

Clinical History

A 60-year-old male with history of right supraorbital and bioccipital headaches, as well as right Horner's syndrome.

Findings

The T1-weighted axial study (Fig. 20A) demonstrates a high signal ring around the flow void of the right internal carotid artery; the lumen exhibits a narrower low signal flow void (*arrow*) than the contralateral (left) channel. The 3D time-of-flight MRA sequence (Fig. 20B) shows an apparent widening of the carotid channel on the right, as compared to the left, in the region of the subpetrous carotid. The targeted reconstruction of this vessel in a slightly different projection (Fig. 20C) shows that the internal carotid artery, in addition to being narrowed below the level of the petrous segment, demonstrates a linear "flap" (*arrowheads*) between the two apparent bright channels.

The intraarterial angiogram (Fig. 20D) verifies the presence of diffuse narrowing of the right internal carotid, particularly at the proximal petrous segment (*arrows*). The follow-up study with 3D time-of-flight MRA (Fig. 20E) demonstrates resolution of the abnormality (obtained 3 months later).

Diagnosis

Right cervical carotid artery dissection.

Discussion

Dissection of the cervical carotid artery occurs from a tear of the intimal lining, which allows deflection of blood into the wall of the vessel. This narrows the vessel lumen and predisposes to turbulence, clot formation, and even vascular occlusion. Although spontaneous resolution of this process can occur (in approximately 68% of the cases), embolic stroke can be a consequence as well. Anticoagulation is the treatment of choice for the time frame during which resolution occurs.

The MRI/MRA features here are relatively classic. The high signal intensity on the spin-echo image is most likely caused by the presence of methemoglobin in the intramural hemorrhage. The maximum intensity projection (MIP) algorithm sees the bright signal of this mural clot indistinguishable from the bright signal of the enhanced flowing spins in the channel, and assumes that both represent the vessel, resulting in the widening shown. However, the actual flap is discerned on the MIP image, and when one takes into account the findings on the spin-echo axial image, the appropriate diagnosis is readily made. The intraarterial angiogram does not demonstrate the false lumen, which contains no flow (thus no contrast), and verifies the narrowed flowing lumen. This study documents MRI/MRA's ability not only to detect cervical carotid dissection, but to follow the patient through its resolution without the need for subsequent invasive angiography.

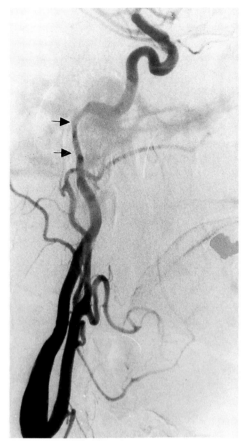 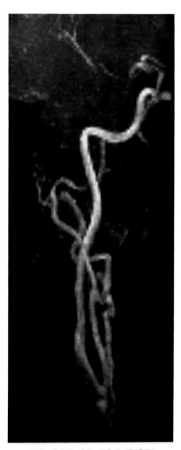

FIG. 20D. Intraarterial DSA RCA.　　　　FIG. 20E. 3D TOF (FISP)
　　　　　　　　　　　　　　　　　　　　40/7/30°.

46

References

1. Edelman RR, Mattle HP, et al. MR Angiography. *AJR* 1990;154:937–946.
2. Goldberg HI, Grossman RI, et al. Cervical internal carotid artery dissecting hemorrhage: diagnosis using MR. *Radiology* 1986;158:157–161.
3. Brugieres P, et al. Magnetic resonance imaging in the exploration of dissection of the internal carotid artery. *J Neuroradiol* 1989;16:1–10.
4. Gelbert F, Assouline E, et al. MRI in spontaneous dissection of the vertebral and carotid arteries. *Neuroradiology* 1991;33:111–113.
5. Nguyen Bui L, Brant-Zawadzki M, et al. MR angiography of cervico-cranial dissection. *Stroke* 1993;24:126–131.

Submitted by: Michael Brant-Zawadzki, M.D., F.A.C.R., Hoag Memorial Hospital, Newport Beach, California; Michael Brant-Zawadzki, M.D., F.A.C.R., Senior Editor.

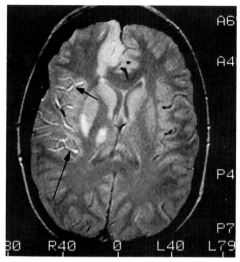

FIG. 21A. SE 2200/30.

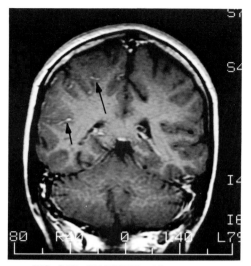

FIG. 21B. SE 500/20 with contrast.

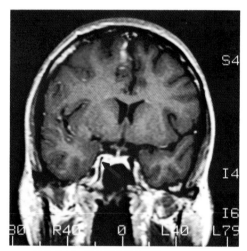

FIG. 21C. SE 500/20 with contrast.

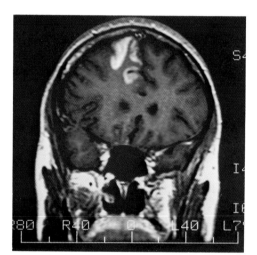

FIG. 21D. SE 500/20 with contrast.

Clinical History

A 38-year-old female presents with sudden neck pain and left hemiparesis.

Findings

Axial proton density image (Fig. 21A) shows abnormal signal intensity in the right basal ganglia and anterior cerebral artery (ACA) distribution. Note the loss of normal flow void of the right middle cerebral artery (MCA) (Fig. 21A, *arrows*). Gadolinium (Gd)-DTPA shows intravascular enhancement of the distal right MCA branches (Fig. 21B, *arrows*), diminutive right internal carotid artery (ICA) diameter (Fig. 21C, *arrow*) and gyriform enhancement of the right frontal lobe (Fig. 21D). Right common carotid angiogram demonstrates a right ICA with decreased caliber and complete occlusion just above the level of the ophthalmic artery (Fig. 21E, *arrow*).

Diagnosis

Spontaneous dissection of the right ICA with complete intracranial occlusion.

Discussion

Intravascular enhancement can be seen as one of the earliest signs of an acute infarct, which can resolve after 1 week post-ictus (1–3).

Intravascular enhancement can be seen in 92% of cases of stroke (1). Blood-brain barrier breakdown and parenchymal enhancement follows the arterial slow flow findings of Gd-DTPA signal replacement of arterial flow void.

References

1. Elster AD, Moody DM. Early cerebral infarction: gadopentetate dimeglumine enhancement. *Radiology* 1990;177:627–632.
2. Sato A, Takahashi S, Soma Y, et al. Cerebral infarction: early detection by means of contrast-enhanced cerebral arteries at MR imaging. *Radiology* 1991;178:433–439.
3. Crain MR, Yuh WTC, Greene GM, et al. Cerebral ischemia: evaluation with contrast-enhanced MR imaging. *AJNR* 1991;12:631–639.

Submitted by: Orest B. Boyko, M.D., Ph.D., Duke University Medical Center, Durham, North Carolina; Michael Brant-Zawadzki, M.D., F.A.C.R., Senior Editor.

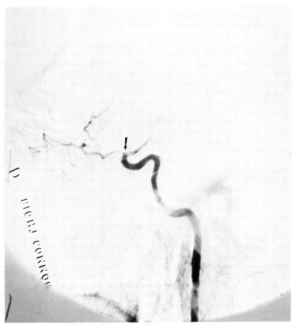

FIG. 21E. Conventional lateral RCCA angiogram.

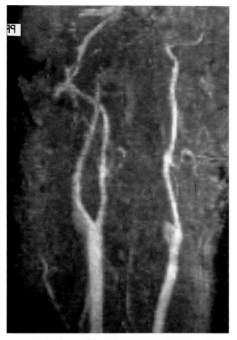

FIG. 22A. 3D TOF (FISP) 40/7/15°.

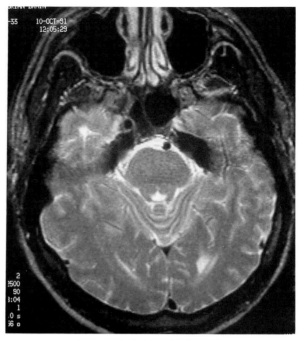

FIG. 22B. Axial SE 2500/90.

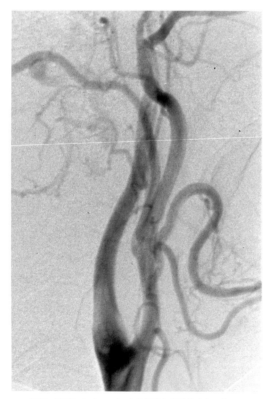

FIG. 22C. Intraarterial DSA RCA injection.

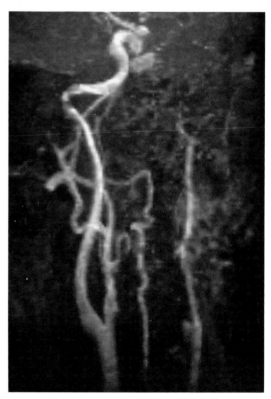

FIG. 22D. 3D TOF (FISP) 40/7/15°.

Clinical History

A 58-year-old male with known left carotid occlusion now presents with drastically altered mental status following several episodes of syncope. Patient is on Cafergot for migraine prophylaxis.

Findings

The initial cervical MRA study (Fig. 22A) demonstrates occlusion of the left carotid artery. The right internal carotid artery shows narrowing and poor definition at the skull base.

Conventional MR image (Fig. 22B) demonstrates loss of signal void in the left carotid artery siphon; normal signal void is seen on the right.

Diagnosis

Right internal carotid artery dissection, status postocclusion of left internal carotid artery.

Discussion

The intraarterial angiogram (Fig. 22C) verifies the dissection of the right internal carotid artery. This patient was placed on anticoagulants and the follow-up MR angiogram demonstrates partial resolution of the dissection (Fig. 22D). He went on to a full recovery and has been maintained on warfarin.

Cafergot (ergotamine tartrate and caffeine) is an anti-migraine medication that predisposes to vascular spasm and potentially dissection. The patient's history obtained subsequently was that he was excessively using the Cafergot. Presumably, the left carotid artery obstruction was also on the basis of dissection. This case demonstrates the utility of MR angiographic studies as a noninvasive follow-up examination.

References

1. Nguyen Bui L, Brant-Zawadzki M, et al. MR angiography of cervicocranial dissection. *Stroke* 1993;24:126–131.
2. Sue D, Brant-Zawadzki M, Chance J. Dissection of cranial arteries in the neck: correlation of MRI and arteriography. *Neuroradiology* 1992;34:273–278.
3. Brant-Zawadzki M, Gillan G. Extracranial carotid magnetic resonance angiography. *Cardiovasc Intervent Radiol* 1992;15:82–90.
4. Wagle WA, Dumoulin CL, et al. 3DFT MR angiography of carotid and basilar arteries. *AJNR* 1989;10:911–919.

Submitted by: Michael Brant-Zawadzki, M.D., F.A.C.R., Hoag Memorial Hospital, Newport Beach, California; Michael Brant-Zawadzki, M.D., F.A.C.R., Senior Editor.

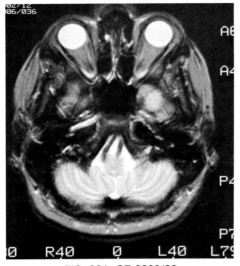

FIG. 23A. SE 2800/80.

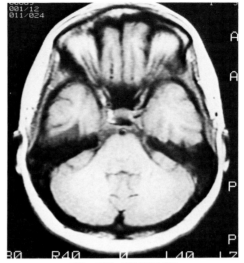

FIG. 23B. SE 500/20.

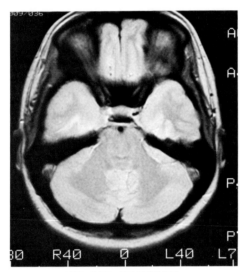

FIG. 23C. SE 2800/30.

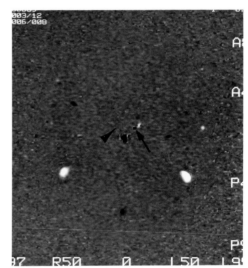

FIG. 23D. 2D PC MRA (24/14; 45° flip angle).

Clinical History

A 32-year-old female with right neck pain and transient ischemic attacks.

Findings

Axial T2-weighted spin-echo image (Fig. 23A) shows signal (lack of flow void) in the horizontal portion of the right internal carotid artery (RICA). The right cavernous ICA shows luminal signal intensity on T1-weighted (Fig. 23B) and proton density (Fig. 23C) images. Axial single slice 2D phase contrast (PC) magnetic resonance angiography (MRA) phase image (Fig. 23D) confirms no flow in the RICA (Fig. 23D, *arrowhead*) but flow in a diminutive LICA (Fig. 23D, *arrow*). Conventional right common carotid artery (CCA) angiogram shows a tapered ICA (Fig. 23E, *arrowheads*) with distal occlusion of the intracranial portion of the RICA.

Diagnosis

Spontaneous dissection of the RICA (with total occlusion) and the LICA.

Discussion

Cervical carotid artery disease can manifest itself as a loss of normal flow void on intracranial spin-echo MR imaging and complete loss of intracranial flow void can correlate with total occlusion of the cervical ICA as demonstrated by this case (1). Angiography may still be required to separate slow flow from total occlusion (2). The presence of normal flow void in the intracranial portion of an ICA does not exclude significant compromise of the cervical segment of the ICA (2). Phase imaging may be helpful in distinguishing signal from thrombus or slow flow (3). In this case the diminutive LICA (Fig. 23D) correlated on conventional angiography with spontaneous dissection and partial occlusion.

References

1. Heinz ER, Yeates AE, Djang WT. Significant extracranial carotid stenosis: detection on routine cerebral MR images. *Radiology* 1989;170:843–848.
2. Brant-Zawadzki M. Routine MR imaging of the internal carotid artery siphon: angiographic correlation with cervical carotid lesions. *AJNR* 1990;11:467–471.
3. Nadel L, Braun IF, Kraft KA, et al. Intracranial vascular abnormalities: value of MR phase imaging to distinguish thrombus from flowing blood. *AJNR* 1991;11:1133–1140.

Submitted by: Orest B. Boyko, M.D., Ph.D., Duke University Medical Center, Durham, North Carolina; Michael Brant-Zawadzki, M.D., F.A.C.R., Senior Editor.

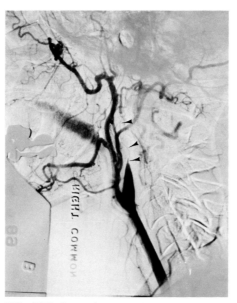

FIG. 23E. Lateral conventional right common carotid angiogram.

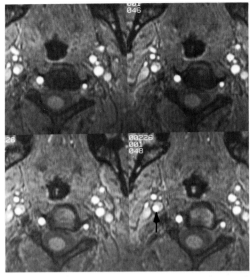

FIG. 24A. MRA 3D TOF gradient-refocused 36/16, no saturation.

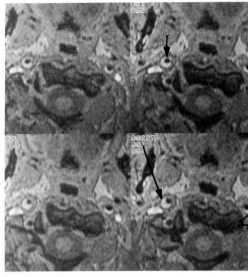

FIG. 24B. MRA 3D TOF gradient-refocused 36/16, with saturation.

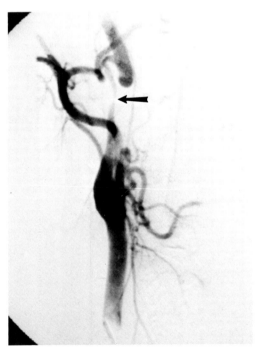

FIG. 24C. Conventional angiogram R ICA.

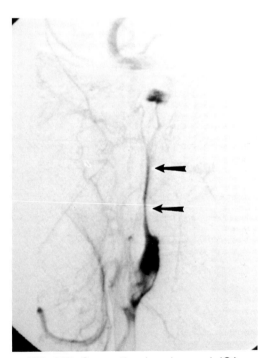

FIG. 24D. Conventional angiogram L ICA.

Clinical History

A 36-year-old male presents with stroke.

Findings

Axial partition images of 3D time-of-flight (TOF) magnetic resonance angiography (MRA) without saturation pulse application shows a narrowed hyperintense true lumen (Fig. 24A, *short arrow*) of the right cervical internal carotid artery (ICA), repeat 3D TOF with application of a saturation pulse reveals a narrowed arterial lumen of the right internal carotid (Fig. 24B, *short arrow*). The signal intensity of the false lumen remains hyperintense (Fig. 24B, *long arrow*). Because the dissection twists in a helical fashion, it is lateral to the true arterial lumen on images in the higher cervical region (Fig. 24B). Incidental note is made of hyperintense dissection of the left internal carotid arterial wall (Fig. 24B, *open arrowhead*). Conventional angiogram of the right ICA confirms narrowed arterial lumen and dissection (Fig. 24C, *arrow*). Conventional angiogram of the left ICA also shows dissection (Fig. 24D, *arrows*).

Diagnosis

Bilateral spontaneous carotid artery dissection.

Discussion

Conventional angiography demonstrates a narrowed lumen in nonocclusive carotid artery dissection (1,2). This case illustrates that the narrowed residual lumen can be shown by 3D TOF MRA using as an adjunct a saturation pulse (2,3). The narrowed arterial lumen has hyperintense signal on nonsaturated images and hyperintense signal on the saturated images. The dissection itself appears hyperintense with or without saturation pulses. MRA partition images allow for excellent visualization of the arterial wall dissection, which cannot be seen on conventional angiograms. The dissection appears semilunar in configuration and "rotates" in a helical fashion around the true lumen.

References

1. Wagle WA. Neuroradiology. In: Joynt RJ. *Clinical neurology.* Philadelphia: Lippincott, 1991.
2. Wagle WA, Dumoulin CL, Souza SP, et al. 3DFT MR angiography of carotid and basilar arteries. *AJNR* 1989;10:911–919.
3. Dumoulin CL, Cline HE, Souza SP, et al. Three dimensional time-of-flight magnetic resonance angiography using spin saturation. *Magn Reson Med* 1989;11:35–46.

Submitted by: William A. Wagle, M.D., Albany Medical Center, Albany, New York; Michael Brant-Zawadzki, M.D., F.A.C.R., Senior Editor.

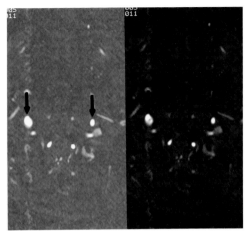

FIG. 25A. 2D PC MRA, gradient-refocused 33/8.

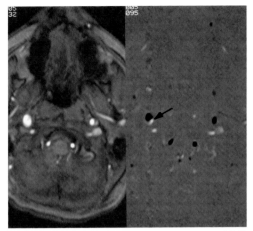

FIG. 25B. 2D PC MRA, gradient-refocused 33/8.

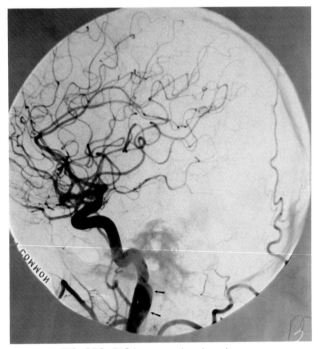

FIG. 25C. RICA conventional angiogram.

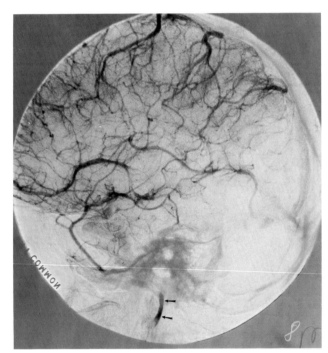

FIG. 25D. RICA conventional angiogram.

Clinical History

A 40-year-old male with right ptosis, miosis, and facial pain but without anhidrosis. Past history of cervical neck trauma 3 years previous.

Findings

Axial 2D phase contrast (PC) magnetic resonance angiography (MRA) speed image at the cervical spine level of C1-C2 demonstrates asymmetry of vessel caliber of the right internal carotid artery (RICA) compared to the left ICA (Fig. 25A, *left, arrows*). Note by changing the window/level setting from 2309/370 to 3310/1050 (Fig. 25A, *right*) it is more apparent that the RICA has a "double lumen" appearance with different signal intensities. The less intense signal in the medial posterior lumen represents slower flow. Further 2D PC MRA images, including the magnitude (Fig. 25B) and phase images (Fig. 25B), show asymmetry of caliber of the RICA compared to the normal LICA. Note on the phase image (Fig. 25B, *right*) that both ICAs and vertebral arteries have dark pixels indicating that these four vessels have similar flow velocity and direction. The medial/posterior lumen (Fig. 25B, *right, arrow*) demonstrates bright pixels indicating that the velocity and/or direction is markedly different in this lumen than the normal arteries at a velocity-encoding (VENC) value of 60 cm/sec. Conventional angiography confirms during the arterial injection a posterior outpouching of the RICA at C1/2 (Fig. 25C, *arrows*). Delayed angiographic image capturing the venous phase shows (Fig. 25D, *arrows*) delayed contrast (slow flow) in the pseudoaneurysm.

Diagnosis

Right internal carotid artery dissecting aneurysm with paratrigeminal syndrome of Raeder.

Discussion

The clinical syndrome described by Raeder (1) consisted of ocular sympathetic paralysis (ptosis and miosis) caused by involvement of the sympathetic fibers in the wall of ICA. Raeder's syndrome has only the ocular findings of Horner's syndrome and there is no loss of sweating on the affected side of the face because these fibers travel with the external carotid artery. The facial pain can be throbbing and intense, felt behind the eye. Thus, an intracranial aneurysm or retro-orbital tumor can be considered in the clinical differential diagnosis.

This case illustrates that 2D PC MRA is sensitive to marked difference in flow velocity (as well as direction), accounting for the difference in signal intensity in the pseudoaneurysm of the false lumen of the dissection (Fig. 25B, *right, arrow*).

References

1. Raeder JB. "Paratrigeminal" paralysis of oculopapillary sympathetic. *Brain* 1924;47:149.
2. Turski P, Bernstein M, Boyko O, et al. *Vascular magnetic resonance imaging.* General Electric Medical Systems, Milwaukee, WI, 1990, 25–37.

Submitted by: Orest B. Boyko, M.D., Ph.D., Duke University Medical Center, Durham, North Carolina; Michael Brant-Zawadzki, M.D., F.A.C.R., Senior Editor.

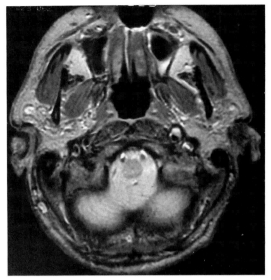

FIG. 26A. Axial SE 2800/30.

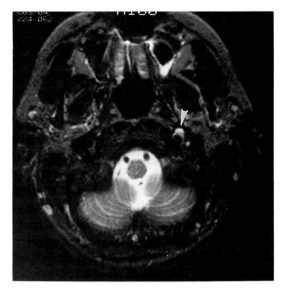

FIG. 26B. Axial SE 2800/90.

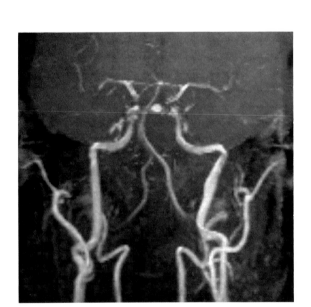

FIG. 26C. 3D TOF (FISP) 40/7/25°.

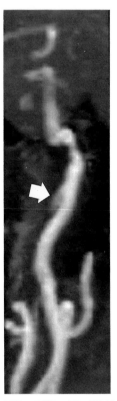

FIG. 26D. 3D TOF (FISP) 40/7/25°.

Clinical History

A 47-year-old male with a 10-day history of left temporal headache, and chronic hypertension.

Findings

The dual echo T2-weighted axial sequence (Figs. 26A and B) demonstrates the normal flow void of the left carotid artery to be surrounded by high signal intensity subjacent to the cranial vault. This is particularly well shown on the second echo (Fig. 26B, *arrowhead*). The 3D time-of-flight MR angiographic study utilizing maximum intensity pixel (MIP) reconstructions (Fig. 26C) demonstrates asymmetry of the subcranial carotid arteries. Selective MIP image (Fig. 26D) of the left carotid artery demonstrates a focal ectasia (*arrow*) of the vessel, as well as some irregularity.

Diagnosis

Dissecting aneurysm of left internal carotid artery.

Discussion

Cervical carotid dissection can produce narrowing as well as focal ectasia to the point of pseudoaneurysm formation. This is an example of such a case. Note that the intraarterial angiogram (Fig. 26E) defines the morphology of the aneurysmal component to better advantage. This patient was placed on anticoagulants and followed noninvasively with MR angiography until resolution.

References

1. Sue DE, Brant-Zawadzki MN, Chance J. Dissection of cranial arteries in the neck: correlation of MRI and arteriography. *Neuroradiology* 1992;34:273–278.
2. Nguyen Bui L, Brant-Zawadzki M, Verghese P, et al. MR angiography of cervico-cranial dissection. *Stroke* 1993;24:126–131.
3. Bradac GB, Kaernbach A, et al. Spontaneous dissecting aneurysm of cervical arteries. *Neuroradiology* 1981;21:149–154.

Submitted by: Michael Brant-Zawadzki, M.D., F.A.C.R., Hoag Memorial Hospital, Newport Beach, California; Michael Brant-Zawadzki, M.D., F.A.C.R., Senior Editor.

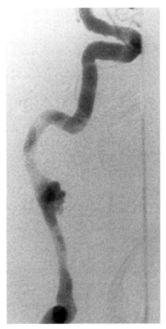

FIG. 26E. Intraarterial DSA LCA.

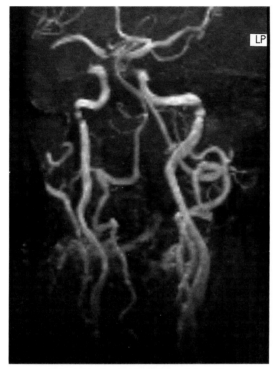

FIG. 27A. 3D TOF (FISP) 40/7/15°.

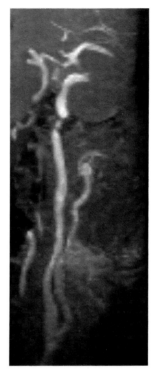

FIG. 27B. 3D TOF (FISP) 40/7/15°.

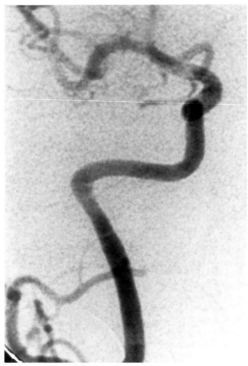

FIG. 27C. Intracranial DSA RCA.

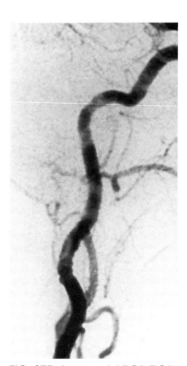

FIG. 27D. Intracranial DSA RCA.

Clinical History

A 60-year-old female with Horner's syndrome.

Findings

The 3D time-of-flight magnetic resonance angiogram (MRA) (Fig. 27A) of the cervicocranial region demonstrates defects in the petrous portions of both carotid arteries. These are band-like defects, occurring at the acute turn of the carotid in the petrous segment. The more proximal internal carotid arteries extending from the bifurcation are grossly unremarkable.

Selected (MRA) view of the right internal carotid artery (Fig. 27B) shows perhaps slight narrowing in the proximal segment of the cervical internal carotid artery, but no focal defects are discernible.

The intraarterial angiogram (Fig. 27C) demonstrates no evidence of abnormality in the petrous segment of the internal carotid artery. However, there is an accordion-like defect of the lumen at the cervical carotid level consistent with fibromuscular hyperplasia (Fig. 27D).

Diagnosis

False-positive MRA for bilateral carotid dissection or stenosis in the petrous segment: false-negative MRA for fibromuscular disease.

Discussion

As shown in Case 19, the presence of narrowing and irregularity in the petrous portion of the carotid artery in a patient with Horner's syndrome suggests the diagnosis of dissection. However, this site is also one where magnetic susceptibility effects of the bone–air interfaces and turbulence due to the acute bend of the carotid contribute to such "defects." The symmetry of the findings is a clue to the "defects" being artifactual.

Fibromuscular disease is a causative lesion for transient ischemic attacks. The fact that MR angiography may not detect subtle intimal fibromuscular disease, as in this case, again indicates that in patients who have clear-cut symptoms of cerebral ischemia, and in whom MR angiography does not explain such symptoms, intraarterial angiography is still necessary as the "gold standard." Incidentally, fibromuscular disease also is one of the lesions that predisposes to dissection. It can be a familial disorder, and it can affect both cervical and vertebral arteries. Typically it is seen at the higher levels of the carotid and vertebral course.

References

1. Anderson CM, Saloner D, et al. Artifacts in maximum-intensity-projection display of MR angiograms. *AJR* 1990;154:623–629.
2. Brant-Zawadzki MN, Gillan G. Extracranial carotid magnetic resonance angiography. *Cardiovasc Intervent Radiol* 1992;15:82–90.
3. Sandok BA. Fibromuscular dysplasia of the internal carotid artery. *Neurol Clin* 1983;1(1).
4. Mettinger KL, Ericson K. Fibromuscular dysplasia and the brain. *Stroke* 1982;13(1).
5. Nguyen Bui L, Brant-Zawadzki M, et al. MR angiography of cervico-cranial dissection. *Stroke* 1993;24:126–131.

Submitted by: Michael Brant-Zawadzki, M.D., F.A.C.R., Hoag Memorial Hospital, Newport Beach, California; Michael Brant-Zawadzki, M.D., F.A.C.R., Senior Editor.

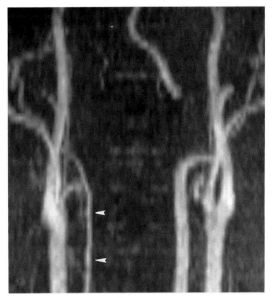

FIG. 28A. 2D TOF (FLASH) 38/9/30°.

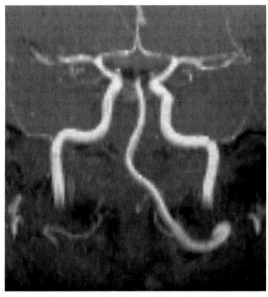

FIG. 28B. 3D TOF (FISP) 40/7/15°.

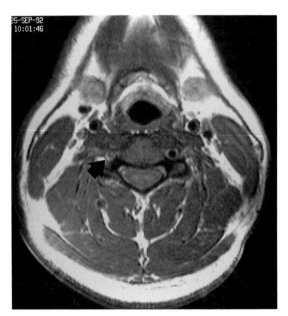

FIG. 28C. Axial SE 8000/22.

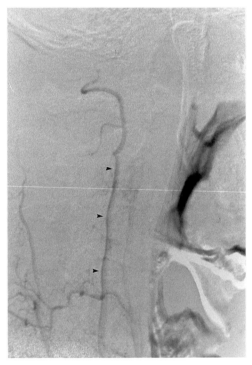

FIG. 28D. Intraarterial DSA LSA.

Clinical History

A 32-year-old male with sudden syncopal episode, status post–motor vehicle accident and chiropractic manipulation.

Findings

The MR examination of the brain was normal. The MR angiogram of the cervicocranial vasculature demonstrates relative hypoplasia of the right vertebral (Fig. 28A, *arrowheads*) artery and loss of contiguity from the distal vertebral region to the basilar (Fig. 28A) on the 2D, time-of-flight (with traveling saturation pulse). The 3D time-of-flight study obtained at the circle of Willis level verifies the absence of distal right vertebral artery/basilar contiguity (Fig. 28B). The T1-weighted axial image at the C1-2 level (Fig. 28C) demonstrates normal flow void in the left vertebral artery, but the right vertebral artery shows elevation of signal intensity in its wall with no apparent normal flow void (the foramen transversarium was normal in size below this level).

Diagnosis

Right vertebral artery dissection and occlusion.

Discussion

This study demonstrates the occlusive disease of the right vertebral to good advantage. Differentiation between hypoplasia of the vertebral and traumatic dissection is quite difficult based on the images alone. However, the history of recent whiplash-type injury and also chiropractic manipulation should raise the suspicion of vascular trauma, particularly given the presentation of syncope. The intraarterial angiogram (Fig. 28D) demonstrates the rather slow flow up the right vertebral artery (*arrowheads*) from a subclavian injection. Note the transition of caliber at the C1 level beyond which only a trickle of flow into the posterior inferior cerebellar artery is demonstrated.

References

1. Sue DE, Brant-Zawadzki MN, Chance J. Dissection of cranial arteries in the neck: correlation of MRI and arteriography. *Neuroradiology* 1992;34:273–278.
2. Traflet RF, Ashok BR, et al. Vertebral artery dissection after rapid head turning. Abbreviated report. *AJNR* 1989;10:650–651.
3. Mas JL, Bousser MG, et al. Extracranial vertebral artery dissections: a review of 13 cases. *Stroke* 1987;18(6):1037–1047.

Submitted by: Michael Brant-Zawadzki, M.D., F.A.C.R., Hoag Memorial Hospital, Newport Beach, California; Michael Brant-Zawadzki, M.D., F.A.C.R., Senior Editor.

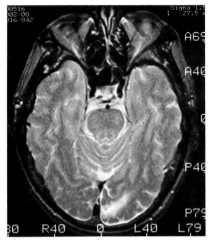

FIG. 29A. SE 2200/80.

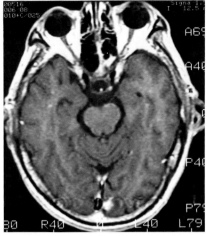

FIG. 29B. Contrast SE 500/20.

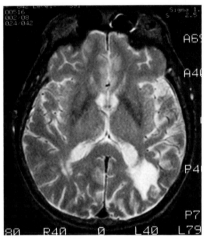

FIG. 29C. SE 2200/80.

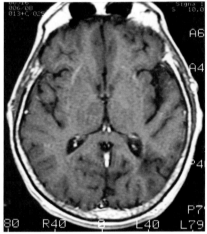

FIG. 29D. Contrast SE 500/20.

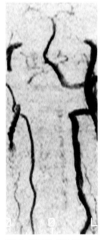
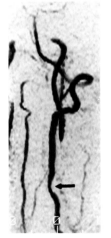

FIG. 29E. 2D TOF
MRA 45/9.

FIG. 29F. 2D TOF
MRA, 45/9.

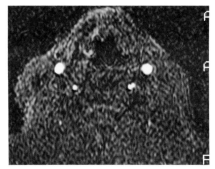 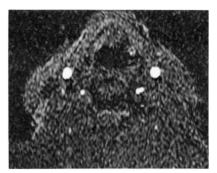

FIG. 29G. 2D TOF MRA, 45/9.　　　FIG. 29H. 2D TOF MRA, 45/9.

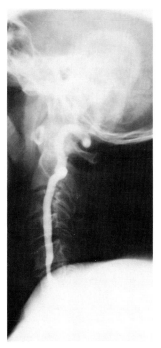

FIG. 29I. Conventional angiogram.

Clinical History

A 64-year-old male with posterior fossa ischemic changes.

Findings

Axial T2-weighted image (Fig. 29A) shows left occipital lobe cortical and subcortical hyperintense signal, with enhancing nodule in the occipital pole seen on T1-weighted image (Fig. 29B). There is a normal flow void in the basilar artery but focal hyperintense signal in the left pons. T2-weighted image at a higher slice (Fig. 29C) reveals subcortical white matter hyperintense signal sparing the subcortical U-fibers and no enhancement (Fig. 29D). The findings could represent tumor or subacute infarction.

The 2D time-of-flight (TOF) magnetic resonance angiogram (MRA) shows a dominant left vertebral artery with a patent basilar and posterior inferior cerebellar artery. On closer inspection there is compromise of the arterial lumen of the proximal left vertebral artery (Fig. 29E) better seen on oblique views (Fig. 29F, *arrow*). Inspection of the axial partition images (each 1.5 mm in thickness) shows a double lumen contour and flap of the left vertebral artery (Figs. 29G and H) confirming a dissection. The narrowed arterial lumen is confirmed on selective conventional left vertebral artery angiogram (Fig. 29I).

Diagnosis

Chronic left vertebral artery dissection with enhancing left occipital lobe infarct.

Discussion

Enhancing subacute infarct can mimic metastasis, abscess, or glioma. As this case illustrates the source for emboli can also be from the cervical neck. The advantage of 2D TOF MRA (1) is the ability to cover a larger region of interest, as in this case, in a short acquisition (148 1.5-mm partitions covered the region from the top of the basilar artery to near the origin of the vertebral artery here). The demonstration of a flap and the false lumen of the dissection on MRA (where conventional angiography gave no vessel wall information and demonstrated only arterial lumen compromise) helped make the diagnosis here. This case also demonstrates a disadvantage to MRA where there is artifactual signal dropout of the right vertebral artery because of its small size and lower signal intensity (2). Ideal MRA acquisition would have included the origin of the left vertebral artery from the aortic arch.

References

1. Keller PJ, Drayer BP, Fram EK, et al. MR angiography with two-dimensional acquisition and three-dimensional display-work in progress. *Radiology* 1989;173:527–532.
2. Anderson CM, Saloner D, Tsuruda JS, et al. Artifacts in maximum-intensity-projection display of MR angiograms. *AJR* 1990;154:623–629.
3. Greselle JF, Zenteno M, Kien P, et al. Spontaneous dissection of the vertebro-basilar system: a study of 18 cases (15 patients). *J Neuroradiol* 1987;14:115–121.

Submitted by: Orest B. Boyko, M.D., Ph.D., Duke University Medical Center, Durham, North Carolina; Michael Brant-Zawadzki, M.D., F.A.C.R., Senior Editor.

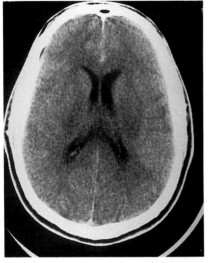

FIG. 30A. Unenhanced axial CT image.

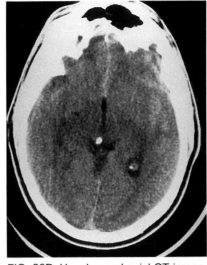

FIG. 30B. Unenhanced axial CT image.

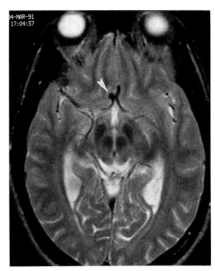

FIG. 30C. Axial SE 2500/90.

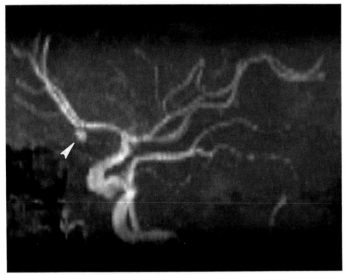

FIG. 30D. 3 TOF (FISP) 40/7/15°.

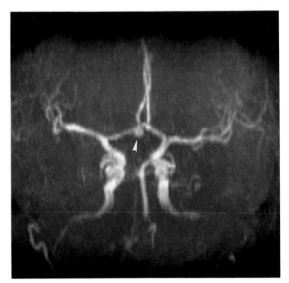

FIG. 30E. 3 TOF (FISP) 40/7/15°.

Clinical History

A 35-year-old male admitted for postcoital seizure.

Findings

Unenhanced CT images (Figs. 30A and B) demonstrate lack of visualization of the cerebral sulci and frontal aspect of the intrahemispheric fissure with subtle hyperdensity seen within these structures. The MR examination (Fig. 30C) obtained immediately afterward does not demonstrate the subarachnoid blood; however, it does depict the presence of a focal region of flow void at the level of the anterior communicating artery (*arrowhead*). The subsequent 3D time-of-flight MR angiogram (Fig. 30D and E) verifies the presence of the aneurysm at the anterior communicating artery level, just to the right of midline (*arrowheads*). The intraarterial angiogram study (Fig. 30F) shows the neck of the aneurysm actually originating at the junction of the right anterior cerebral and communicating artery region (*arrow*).

Diagnosis

Subarachnoid hemorrhage from anterior communicating artery aneurysm rupture.

Discussion

The definitive tests for clinically suspected subarachnoid hemorrhage is the lumbar puncture. Even CT scanning can miss subarachnoid hemorrhage from aneurysm rupture in up to 10% to 25% of the cases. In this case, subtle findings of subarachnoid bleeding are present on the CT study. MR will miss subarachnoid blood in the acute phase, due to relatively high oxygen tension of the spinal fluid, thus preservation of oxyhemoglobin in the subarachnoid space and lack of typical signal alteration due to bleeding. Nevertheless, MR can show the aneurysm itself, which the CT is less likely to depict. Thus, MR, in conjunction with lumbar puncture, is perhaps the more appropriate choice for evaluating suspected subarachnoid hemorrhage.

The intraarterial angiogram demonstrates its superior spatial resolution for depicting the exact orientation of the aneurysm neck to the parent vessels. Though MRA can provide multiple orientations of the vessels after image acquisition, intraarterial angiography remains the preoperative standard examination for aneurysm management.

References

1. Davis JM, Ploetz J. Cranial computed tomography in subarachnoid hemorrhage: relationship detected by CT and lumbar puncture. *J Comput Assist Tomogr* 1980;4(6):794–796.
2. Ross JS, Masaryk TJ. Intracranial aneurysms: evaluation by MR angiography. *AJR* 1990;155:449–455.
3. Sevick RJ, Tsuruda JS. Three-dimensional time-of-flight MR angiography in the evaluation of cerebral aneurysms. *J Comput Assist Tomogr* 1990;14(6):874–881.
4. Bradley WG, Schnidt PG. Effect of methemoglobin formation on the MR appearance of subarachnoid hemorrhage. *Radiology* 1985;156:99–103.
5. De La Paz RL, New PFJ, et al. NMR imaging of intracranial hemorrhage. *J Comput Assist Tomogr* 1984;8(4):599–607.
6. Kirkwood RJ. Intracranial aneurysm and subarachnoid hemorrhage. In: Kirkwood RJ, ed. *Essentials of neuroimaging.* New York: Churchill-Livingstone, 1990;101–118.

Submitted by: Michael Brant-Zawadzki, M.D., F.A.C.R., Hoag Memorial Hospital, Newport Beach, California; Michael Brant-Zawadzki, M.D., F.A.C.R., Senior Editor.

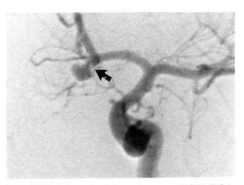

FIG. 30F. Intraarterial angiogram (DSA) RCA.

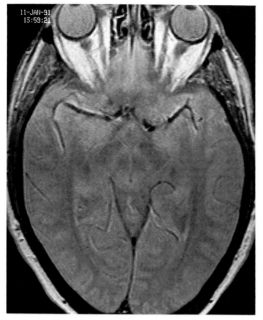

FIG. 31A. Axial SE 2800/22-90.

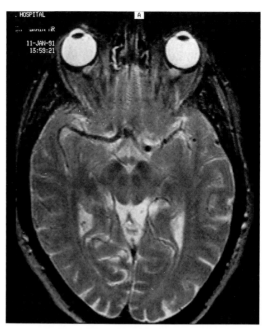

FIG. 31B. Axial SE 2800/22-90.

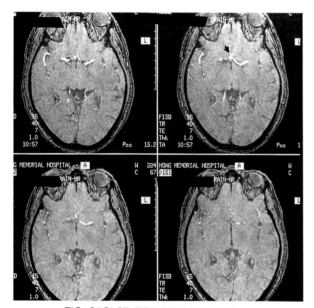

FIG. 31C. 3D TOF FISP 40/7/15°.

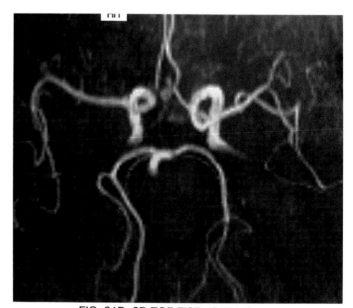

FIG. 31D. 3D TOF FISP 40/7/15°.

Clinical History

A 63-year-old male with sudden onset of the worst headache of his life during defecation.

Findings

The dual echo axial images (Figs. 31A and B) reveal no definite abnormality at the level of the circle of Willis. The rest of the study was unremarkable as well. A 3D time-of-flight angiogram was performed, the partitions of which are shown in Fig. 31C, suggesting a small flow abnormality in the region of the anterior communicating artery (*arrow*). The maximum intensity projection (MIP) algorithm reconstruction shown in Fig. 31D demonstrates a bilobed small outpouching in the anterior communicating artery region on the base projection. This is verified as a bilobed "Mickey Mouse ears" aneurysm on the intraarterial angiographic base view (Fig. 31E).

Diagnosis

Small bilobed aneurysm of anterior communicating artery, at the junction with left anterior cerebral.

Discussion

This study raises the issues of the role of MRI in screening patients with acute subarachnoid hemorrhage. A CT scan is the imaging method of choice for detection of subarachnoid bleeding, although CT has a false-negative rate of 10% to 25%, as documented by the presence of subarachnoid hemorrhage at lumbar puncture. Therefore, a negative CT scan does not obviate the need for lumbar puncture when clinically subarachnoid hemorrhage is suspected. MRI is not as sensitive to the presence of subarachnoid blood for a variety of reasons, including the relatively elevated oxygen tension of spinal fluid (precluding formation of deoxyhemoglobin), spinal fluid pulsations, and possibly other factors. However, MRI with MRA has the potential of detecting even small aneurysms. In this case, the MRA was obtained soon after the physician saw the patient in his office. At this time, his clinical assessment was that the patient had suffered a subarachnoid hemorrhage and the need to identify the site of hemorrhage was paramount. The intraarterial angiogram was performed preoperatively to help verify the findings and exclude the presence of other aneurysms (which can occur with the frequency as high as 20%).

At the current stage of development, MR angiography is insufficient to exclude the presence of small aneurysms in 100% of the cases. Nevertheless, MRA is proving itself to be the most sensitive technique for screening patients noninvasively for the presence of aneurysms. At surgery, the bilobed aneurysm measured approximately 3 and 5 mm for the two lobes.

References

1. Davis JM, Ploetz J. Cranial computed tomography in subarachnoid hemorrhage: relationship detected by CT and lumbar puncture. *J Comput Assist Tomogr* 1980;4(6):794–796.
2. Ross JS, Masaryk TJ. Intracranial aneurysms: evaluation by MR angiography. *AJR* 1990;155:449–455.
3. Sevick RJ, Tsuruda JS. Three-dimensional time-of-flight MR angiography in the evaluation of cerebral aneurysms. *J Comput Assist Tomogr* 1990;14(6):874–881.
4. Bradley WG, Schnidt PG. Effect of methemoglobin formation on the MR appearance of subarachnoid hemorrhage. *Radiology* 1985;156:99–103.
5. De La Paz RL, New PFJ, et al. NMR imaging of intracranial hemorrhage. *J Comput Assist Tomogr* 1984;8(4):599–607.
6. Kirkwood RJ. Intracranial aneurysm and subarachnoid hemorrhage. In: Kirkwood RJ, ed. *Essentials of neuroimaging.* New York: Churchill-Livingstone, 1990;101–118.

Submitted by: Michael Brant-Zawadzki, M.D., F.A.C.R., Hoag Memorial Hospital, Newport Beach, California; Michael Brant-Zawadzki, M.D., F.A.C.R., Senior Editor.

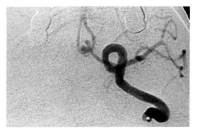

FIG. 31E. Conventional angiogram LCA.

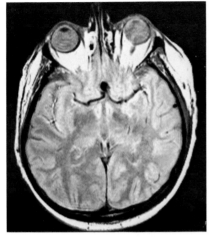

FIG. 32A. SE 2500/22.

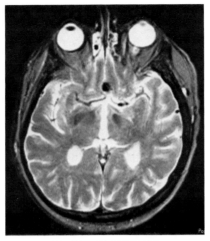

FIG. 32B. SE 2500/90.

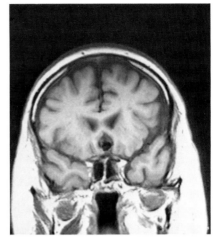

FIG. 32C. SE Coronal SE 600/15.

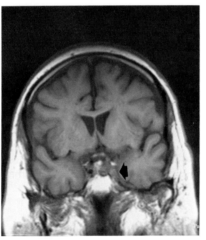

FIG. 32D. Coronal SE 600/15.

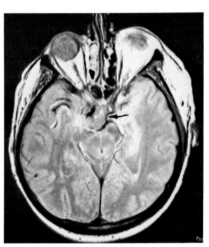

FIG. 32E. SE 2500/22.

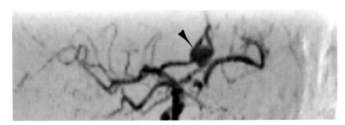

FIG. 32F. Frontal, MRA gradient-refocused 3D TOF.

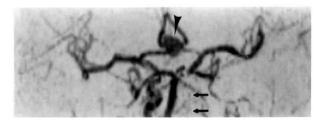

FIG. 32G. Oblique, MRA gradient-refocused 3D TOF.

Clinical History

A 65-year-old male with headache.

Findings

Axial spin density (Fig. 32A) and T2-weighted images (Fig. 32B) show lobular flow void in the interhemispheric fissure in the region of the anterior communicating artery, also visualized on coronal T1-weighted images (Fig. 32C). Lack of flow void is seen on coronal T1-weighted images in the left internal carotid artery (ICA) (Fig. 32D, *arrowhead*). A patent right posterior communicating artery is present (Fig. 32E, *arrow*) indicating collateral flow through the circle of Willis.

The 3D time-of-flight (TOF) magnetic resonance angiography (MRA) reveals in the frontal and oblique projections an anterior communicating aneurysm (Figs. 32F and G, *arrowheads*) and no flow in the petrous and supraclinoid portion of the left ICA (Figs. 32F and G, *arrows*).

Diagnosis

Anterior communicating artery aneurysm, occluded left internal carotid with collateralization through left posterior communicating artery.

Discussion

Of the approximately 20,000 patients whose aneurysms rupture each year, 50% to 60% die within the first 30 days after rupture. The incidence of asymptomatic anterior circulation aneurysms is 1% (1). MRA can provide useful information in imaging aneurysms (2) and vessel patency. Detecting an incomplete circle of Willis, or occlusion of one of the major cranial vessels helps in planning the therapeutic approach.

References

1. Atkinson JLD, Sandt TM, Houser OW, et al. Angiographic frequency of anterior circulation intracranial aneurysms. *J Neurosurg* 1989;70:551–555.
2. Ross JS, Masaryk TJ, Modic MT, et al. Intracranial aneurysms: evaluation by MR angiography. *AJNR* 1990;11:449–456.

Submitted by: Thomas J. Masaryk, M.D., The Cleveland Clinic, Cleveland, Ohio; Michael Brant-Zawadzki, M.D., F.A.C.R., Senior Editor.

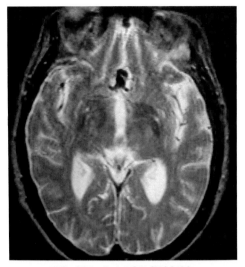

FIG. 33A. Axial SE 2500/90.

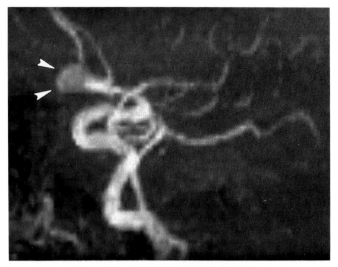

FIG. 33B. 3D TOF (FISP) 40/7/15°.

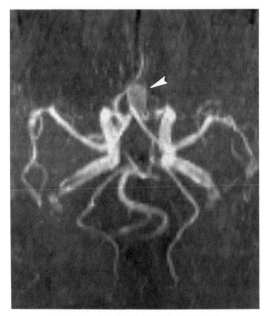

FIG. 33C. 3D TOF (FISP) 40/7/15°.

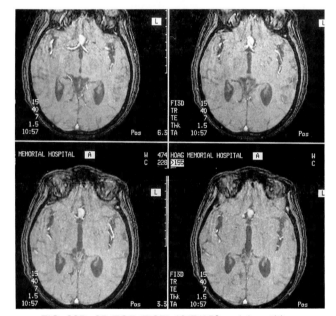

FIG. 33D. 3D TOF (FISP) 40/7/15°, axial partition.

Clinical History

A 73-year-old female with history of headaches whose outside CT examination showed a midline enhancing lesion.

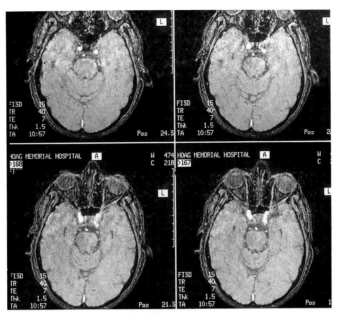

FIG. 33E. 3D TOF (FISP) 40/7/15°, axial partition.

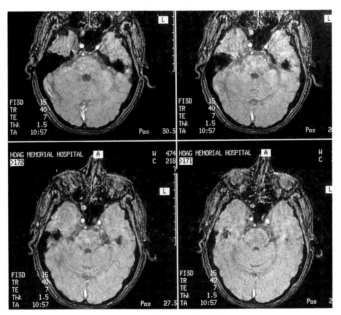

FIG. 33F. 3D TOF (FISP) 40/7/15°, axial partition.

Findings

The T2-weighted image (Fig. 33A) reveals a large focus of signal void adjacent to the interhemispheric fissure, at the level of the anterior communicating artery. The targeted maximum intensity projection (MIP) left lateral and base view images (Figs. 33B and C, respectively) reveal high signal intensity at the level of the anterior communicating artery (*arrows*), which is related more to the junction of the A-1 and A-2 segment of the left anterior cerebral artery. The cavernous and paraclinoid carotid arteries are unremarkable. The partitions (Figs. 33D–F) from the MRA study corroborate these findings. The intraarterial angiogram (Fig. 33G) verifies the presence of a moderately large aneurysm of the left anterior cerebral artery–communicating artery junction region. In addition, a small aneurysm is seen at the genu of the cavernous carotid (*arrow*).

Diagnosis

Anterior communicating artery aneurysm, with second aneurysm of cavernous carotid segment.

Discussion

This case again points out the fact that large aneurysms are usually shown even on conventional MR spin-echo images, with MR angiography showing the patent lumen to good advantage. However, cavernous carotid aneurysms can be missed with MRA. Even with particular attention to the original partitions (1.5 mm thick in this case), MRA was unable to depict the subclinoid carotid artery aneurysm.

The natural history of cavernous carotid segment aneurysms is somewhat more benign. These are less likely to rupture and produce subarachnoid hemorrhage with all of its complications. Rather, the aneurysms tend to grow over time, presenting with ophthalmoplegia or headaches. If they do rupture, the typical lesion produced is a cavernous carotid artery fistula, a lesion more easily treated with today's angiointerventional techniques than the cavernous carotid artery aneurysm itself.

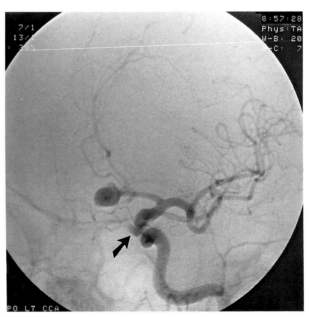

FIG. 33G. Intracranial DSA left carotid injection.

References

1. Ross J, Masaryk TJ, et al. Intracranial aneurysms: evaluation by MR angiography. *AJNR* 1990;11:449–456.
2. Sevick RJ, Tsuruda JS, et al. Three-dimensional time-of-flight MR angiography in the evaluation of cerebral aneurysms. *J Comput Assist Tomogr* 1990;14(6):874–881.
3. Olson WL, Brant-Zawadzki MN, et al. Giant intracranial aneurysms: MR imaging. *Radiology* 1987;163:431–435.

Submitted by: Michael Brant-Zawadzki, M.D., F.A.C.R., Hoag Memorial Hospital, Newport Beach, California; Michael Brant-Zawadzki, M.D., F.A.C.R., Senior Editor.

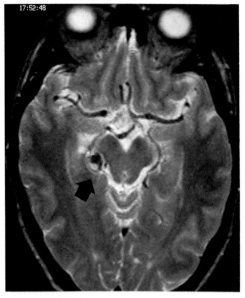

FIG. 34A. Axial SE 2500/90.

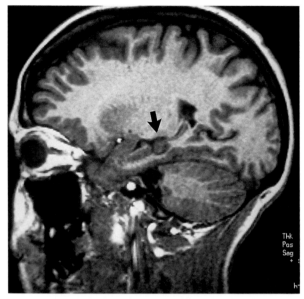

FIG. 34B. 3D sagittal MPRAGE 10/4/12°.

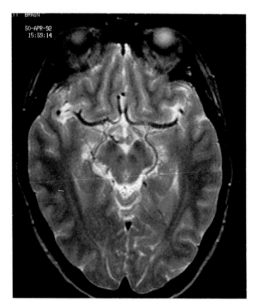

FIG. 34C. Axial SE 2500/90.

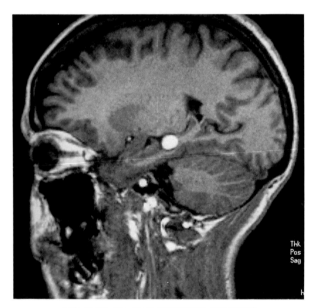

FIG. 34D. Sagittal MPRAGE 10/4/12°.

Clinical History

A 29-year-old female with transient left arm weakness and mild headache.

Findings

The initial MRI scans (Fig. 34A) demonstrates a region of focal low signal intensity in the right ambient cistern or mesiohippocampus (*arrow*). The T1-weighted sagittal image (Fig. 34B) shows this to be a well-circumscribed relatively isointense region (*arrow*). A scan obtained 1 month later demonstrates alteration of signal intensity with high signal now shown in the focus on both the T2- and T1-weighted images (Figs. 34C and D, respectively). Note that the MR angiogram (Fig. 34E) shows that the high signal intensity focus is intimately related to the cerebral vascular structures.

The intraarterial angiogram (Fig. 34F) shows a small outpouching (*arrow*) on the lateral hemispheric branch of the posterior cerebral artery. Nevertheless, the large focus shown on the MRI is not apparent on the intraarterial angiogram. Surgery verified a thrombosed aneurysm at this site.

Diagnosis

Right posterior cerebral artery aneurysm.

Discussion

Surgical planning was made easier by 3D renditions of the MR data set, which utilized both the MR angiographic study and the 3D T1-weighted set of data [a magnetization prepared, gradient recalled turbo-flash sequence (MPRAGE) (Fig. 34G)]. Note the clear demonstration of relationships between the vessels, brain, and the lesion. Also, transparent windows to the abnormality through the scalp (Fig. 34H) and brain surface (Fig. 34I) helped in craniotomy planning.

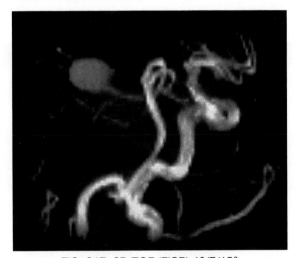

FIG. 34E. 3D TOF (FISP) 40/7/15°.

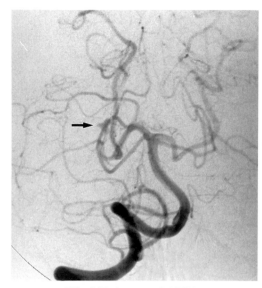

FIG. 34F. Intracranial DSA.

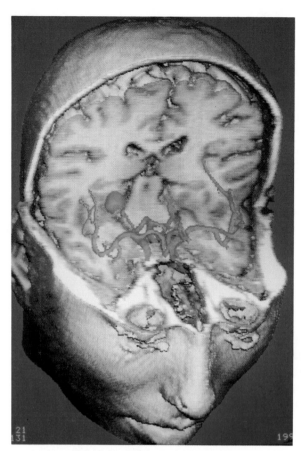

FIG. 34G. 3D surface rendition.

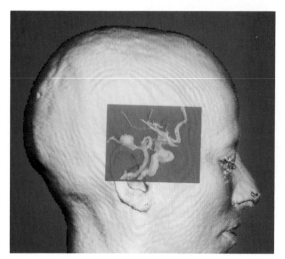

FIG. 34H. 3D surface rendition with transparency overlay.

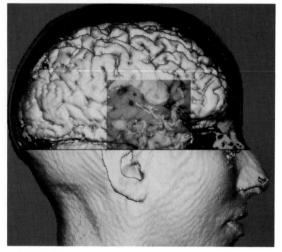

FIG. 34I. 3D surface rendition with transparency overlay.

References

1. Cline HE, Lorensen WE, et al. 3D surface rendered MR images of the brain and its vasculature. *J Comput Assist Tomogr* 1991;15(2):344–351.
2. Bomans M, Karl-Heinz H, et al. Improvement of 3D acquisition and visualization in MRI. *Magn Reson Imaging* 1991;9:597–609.
3. Hu X, Tan K, et al. Three-dimensional magnetic resonance images of the brain: application of neurosurgical planning. *J Neurosurg* 1990;72:433–440.

Submitted by: Michael Brant-Zawadzki, M.D., F.A.C.R., Hoag Memorial Hospital, Newport Beach, California; Michael Brant-Zawadzki, M.D., F.A.C.R., Senior Editor.

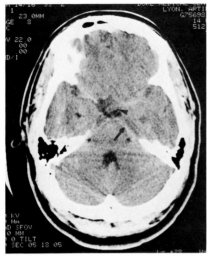

FIG. 35A. Axial non-contrast CT scan.

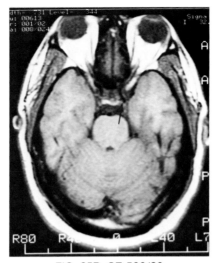

FIG. 35B. SE 500/20.

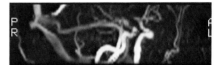

FIG. 35C. 3D PC MRA (36/9; 45° flip angle; VENC 30 cm/sec).

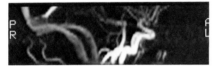

FIG. 35D. 3D PC MRA.

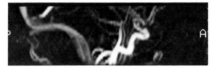

FIG. 35E. 3D PC MRA (180° oblique).

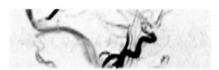

FIG. 35F. 3D PC MRA (180° oblique; video inverted).

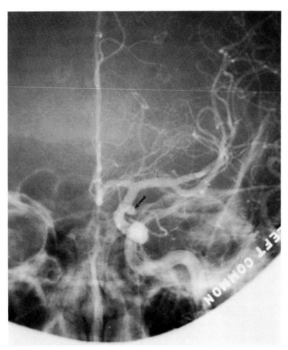

FIG. 35G. AP conventional left CCA angiogram.

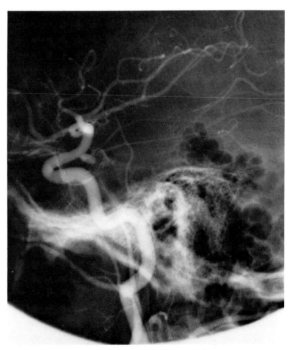

FIG. 35H. Lateral conventional left CCA angiogram.

History

A 24-year-old male presents with the worst headache of his life. Lumbar puncture is positive for subarachnoid hemorrhage (SAH).

Findings

Computed tomography demonstrates questionable left pontine cistern subarachnoid blood (Fig. 35A, *arrow*) and left suprasellar cistern soft tissue density (Fig. 35A, *arrowhead*). T1-weighted image demonstrates no CSF signal intensity abnormality but possibly eccentric flow void of the posterior left supraclinoid internal carotid artery (ICA) (Fig. 35B, *arrow*). T2-weighted images were negative for SAH. The 3D phase contrast (PC) magnetic resonance angiography (MRA) using a velocity encoding (VENC) of 30 cm/sec demonstrates no circle of Willis aneurysm (Figs. 35C–F). Conventional left common carotid artery (CCA) angiogram demonstrates in the anteroposterior (AP) (Fig. 35G) and lateral (Fig. 35H) projection a 3 mm posterior communicating artery (PCoA) aneurysm.

Diagnosis

SAH from a left PCoA aneurysm.

Discussion

This case illustrates that the detection of SAH may be difficult both on CT and MR. Recent encouraging results of detecting SAH by MR have been reported (1). The actual depiction of the aneurysm on spin-echo (SE) images is reported to be up to 54% if 5 mm or larger but 0% if 4 mm or smaller (1). Thinner slices may improve the detection rate, which for CT can be as high as 67% (1). MRA in one series defined 18 of 21 aneurysms (2) but the precise aneurysm neck was not often visualized. Saturation effects from central vortex slow flow or in plane flow can all contribute to the lack of visualization of an aneurysm as well as the choice of flip angle (the greater the flip angle the greater the potential saturation effect), VENC, and slice thickness (the thinner the slice, the less the phase dispersion).

References

1. Satoh S, Kadoya S. Magnetic resonance imaging of subarachnoid hemorrhage. *Neuroradiology* 1990;30:361–366.
2. Ross JS, Masaryk TJ, Modic MT, et al. Intracranial aneurysms: evaluation by MR angiography. *AJNR* 1990;11:449–456.
3. Dumoulin CL, Souza SP, Walker MF, Wagle W. Three-dimensional phase contrast angiography. *Magn Reson Med* 1989;9:139–149.

Submitted by: Orest B. Boyko, M.D., Ph.D., Duke University Medical Center, Durham, North Carolina; Michael Brant-Zawadzki, M.D., F.A.C.R., Senior Editor.

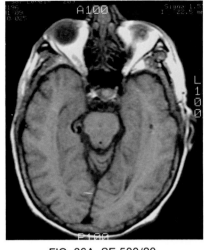

FIG. 36A. SE 500/20.

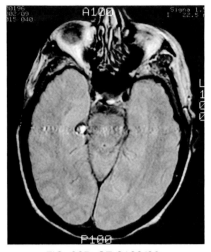

FIG. 36B. SE 2100/30.

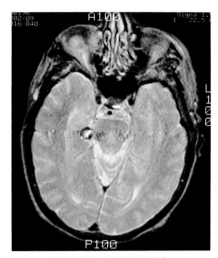

FIG. 36C. SE 2100/80.

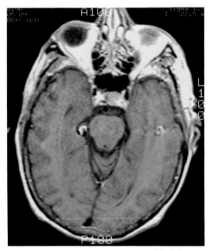

FIG. 36D. Contrast SE 500/20.

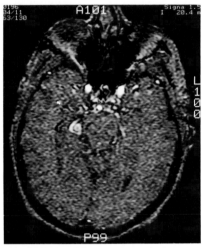

FIG. 36E. 2D TOF MRA, 45/9. 2-D collapsed.

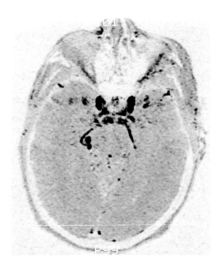

FIG. 36F. 2D TOF MRA, 45/9. 2-D collapsed, video inverted.

Clinical History

A 73-year-old female with past history of carcinoma of the tongue.

Findings

T1-weighted (Fig. 36A) and T2-weighted images (Figs. 36B and C) show an extraaxial mass in the perimesencephalic cistern having peripheral decreased signal intensity representing calcium, blood products, or possibly flow void. Centrally there is signal present and a small focus of flow void. Outside the boundaries of the lesion, in the phase-encoding direction, is the presence of ghosting artifact or smears, indicating that there is flow within the lesion and it is not totally thrombosed (Figs. 36B and C). Contrast T1-weighted image shows gadolinium present within the lesion, indicating slow flow (Fig. 36D). The 2D time-of-flight (TOF) magnetic resonance angiography (MRA) using a superior saturation pulse reveals flow-related enhancement (FRE) in the lesion on 2D collapsed (Figs. 36E and F, video inverted) reprojections.

Diagnosis

Aneurysm of the right posterior cerebral artery.

Discussion

The visualization of ghost artifacts associated with a lesion indicates the presence of pulsatile flow (1). As this case illustrates, complete flow void from time-of-flight or washout effects on spin-echo images may not always accompany the ghost artifacts. These artifacts propagate along the phase-encoding axis, regardless of the direction of flow in the vessel lumen. The artifact appears as bright and dark "smears" but may not exactly replicate the vessel lumen shape. MRA continues to define its role in imaging intracranial cerebral aneurysms (2).

References

1. Spritzer CE, Blinder RA. Vascular applications of magnetic resonance imaging. *Magn Reson Q* 1989;5:205–227.
2. Masaryk TJ, Modic MT, Ross JS, et al. Intracranial circulation: preliminary clinical results with three-dimensional (volume) MR angiography. *Radiology* 1989;171:793–799.

Submitted by: Orest B. Boyko, M.D., Ph.D., Duke University Medical Center, Durham, North Carolina; Michael Brant-Zawadzki, M.D., F.A.C.R., Senior Editor.

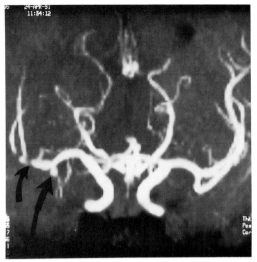

FIG. 37A. 3D TOF (FISP) 35/7/25°.

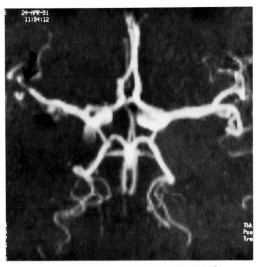

FIG. 37B. 3D TOF (FISP) 35/7/25°.

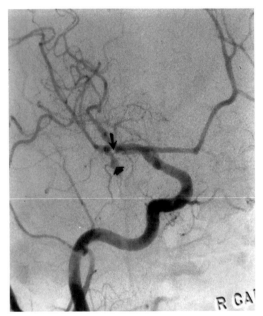

FIG. 37C. Intraarterial DSA RCA injection.

Clinical History

A 26-year-old female IV drug abuser.

Discussion

Two views from an MR angiogram performed with 3D time-of-flight technique demonstrates a small out-pouching (Fig. 37A, *long arrow;* Fig. 37B, *short arrow*) at the right middle cerebral artery trifurcation. Distally, the right middle cerebral artery also shows a focal narrowing (Fig. 37A, *curved arrow;* Fig. 37B, *straight arrow*).

Diagnosis

Mycotic aneurysm.

Discussion

This study again demonstrates the ability of MRA to detect aneurysms distal to the circle of Willis as well as its ability to show stenoses of the major intracranial branches. In this case, intraarterial angiography (Fig. 37C) verified the findings. At surgery (aneurysm—*short arrow,* stenosis—*long arrow*), the mycotic aneurysm was clipped and the middle cerebral artery stenosis was found to be due to a granuloma.

References

1. Heiserman TE, Drayer BP, et al. Intracranial vascular stenosis and occlusion: evaluation with three-dimensional time-of-flight MR angiography. *Radiology* 1992;185:667–673.
2. Masaryk TJ, Modic MT, et al. Intracranial circulation: preliminary clinical results with three-dimensional (volume) MR angiography. *Radiology* 1989;171:793–799.
3. Ross JS, Masaryk TJ, et al. Intracranial aneurysms: evaluation by MR angiography. *AJNR* 1990;11:449–456.
4. Sevick RJ, Tsuruda JS, et al. Three-dimensional time-of-flight MR angiography in the evaluation of cerebral aneurysms. *J Comput Assist Tomogr* 1990;14(6):874–881.

Submitted by: Anton N. Hasso, M.D., F.A.C.R., Loma Linda University School of Medicine, Loma Linda, California; Michael Brant-Zawadzki, M.D., F.A.C.R., Senior Editor.

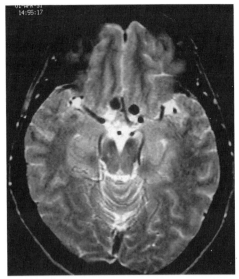

FIG. 38A. Axial SE 2500/90.

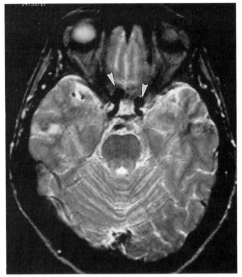

FIG. 38B. Axial SE 2500/90.

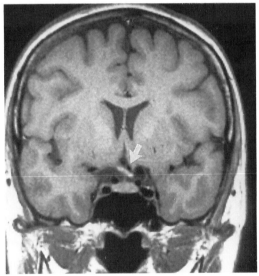

FIG. 38C. Coronal SE 500/15.

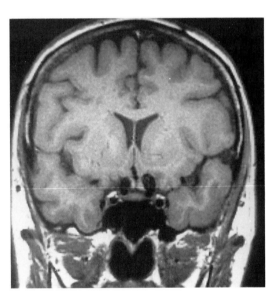

FIG. 38D. Coronal SE 500/15.

Clinical History

A 47-year-old female with visual disturbance and headaches.

Findings

The T2-weighted axial images (Figs. 38A and B) show well-circumscribed foci of signal void in relation to the supraclinoid carotid artery siphons (Fig. 38B, *arrowheads*). The coronal T1-weighted images (Figs. 38C–E) demonstrate the relationship of these abnormal vascular structures to the optic chiasm. Note the leftward tilt of the chiasm (Fig. 38C, *arrow*) and the close relationship of the abnormal vascular structures to the optic nerves themselves on the more anterior slices (Figs. 38D and E). The 3D time-of-flight angiogram, base view (Fig. 38F), verifies the presence of mirror aneurysms at the junction of the supraclinoid carotid and anterior cerebral (A-1) segments.

Diagnosis

Bilateral supraclinoid aneurysms.

Discussion

This patient's referral was through an ophthalmologist, for deteriorating vision. The mass effect of aneurysms on the optic nerves was the etiology. Other common ophthalmologic syndromes with intracranial artery aneurysms include third nerve palsy from posterior communicating artery aneurysms, as well as sixth nerve palsy (or multiple ophthalmic nerve palsies) from cavernous carotid aneurysms.

References

1. Ross JS, Masaryk TJ, et al. Intracranial aneurysms: evaluation by MR angiography. *AJNR* 1990;11:449–456.
2. Atlas, SW. Intracranial vascular malformations and aneurysms. In: Atlas SW, ed. *Magnetic resonance imaging of the brain and spine.* New York: Raven Press, 1991;379–409.
3. Kwan ESK, Laucilla M, et al. A cliniconeuroradiologic approach to third nerve palsies. *AJNR* 1987;8:459–468.

Submitted by: Michael Brant-Zawadzki, M.D., F.A.C.R., Hoag Memorial Hospital, Newport Beach, California; Michael Brant-Zawadzki, M.D., F.A.C.R., Senior Editor.

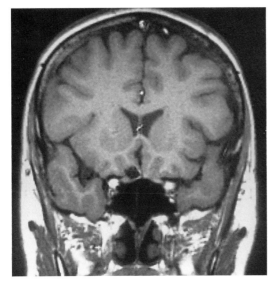

FIG. 38E. Coronal SE 500/15.

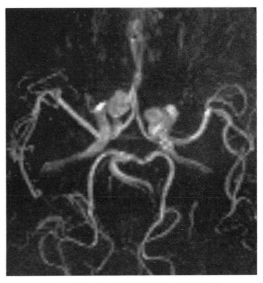

FIG. 38F. 3D TOF (FISP) 40/7/15°.

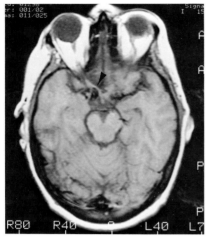

FIG. 39A. SE 500/20.

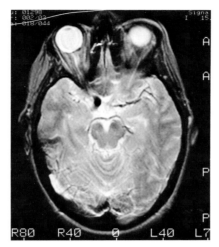

FIG. 39B. SE 2500/80.

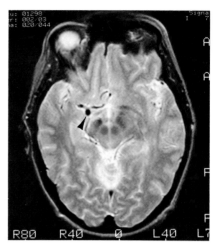

FIG. 39C. SE 2500/80.

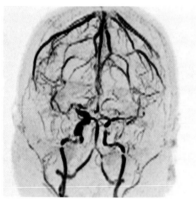

FIG. 39D. 2D TOF MRA AP view (55/9; 60 deg flip angle).

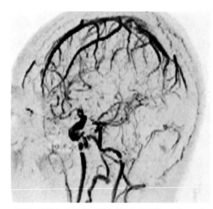

FIG. 39E. 2D TOF MRA (50° oblique).

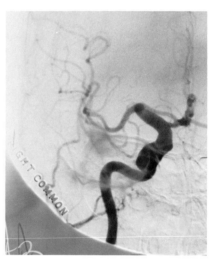

FIG. 39F. Conventional RCCA angiogram (AP view).

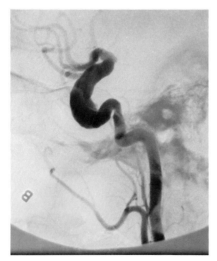

FIG. 39G. Conventional RCCA angiogram (lateral view).

Clinical History

A 48-year-old female complains of right eye blindness.

Findings

T1-weighted MR image shows the right optic nerve displaced medially (Fig. 39A, *arrowhead*) by a lesion having hypointense signal (flow void). T2-weighted image (Fig. 39B) confirms the flow void and raises a question of a middle cerebral artery (MCA) aneurysm (Fig. 39C, *arrowhead*).

The 2D time-of-flight (TOF) magnetic resonance angiography (MRA) 3D reprojection images in the anteroposterior (AP) and oblique projection (Figs. 39D and E) demonstrate a fusiform aneurysmal expansion of the midsiphon and intracavernous portion of the right internal carotid artery (ICA) extending to its intracranial bifurcation. Conventional angiogram of a right common carotid artery injection confirms the finding as seen in the AP (Fig. 39F) and lateral view (Fig. 39G).

Diagnosis

Fusiform aneurysm of the right ICA with optic nerve compression.

Discussion

The 2D TOF MRA (1) provides excellent sensitivity to arterial (fast) and venous (slow) flow. Note that even with the use of a superior saturation pulse, only venous flow in the superior to inferior direction (transverse, sigmoid, and posterior superior sagittal venous sinuses) are saturated and thus not visualized. The anterior superior sagittal venous sinus and the superficial cortical veins flow inferior to superior (analogous to the flow direction in the arteries) and are visualized even in the presence of a superior saturation pulse.

Reference

1. Keller PJ, Drayer BP, Fram EK, et al. MR angiography with two-dimensional acquisition and three dimensional display—work in progress. *Radiology* 1989;173:527–532.

Submitted by: Orest B. Boyko, M.D., Ph.D., Duke University Medical Center, Durham, North Carolina; Michael Brant-Zawadzki, M.D., F.A.C.R., Senior Editor.

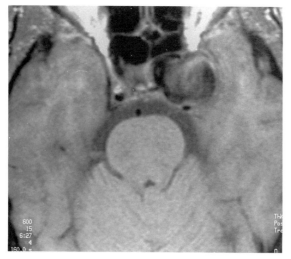

FIG. 40A. Axial SE 600/15.

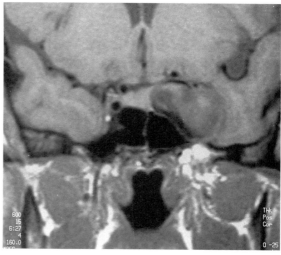

FIG. 40B. Coronal SE 600/15.

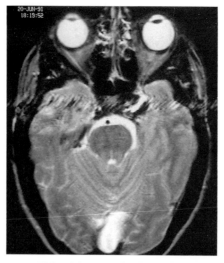

FIG. 40C. Axial SE 2,500/90.

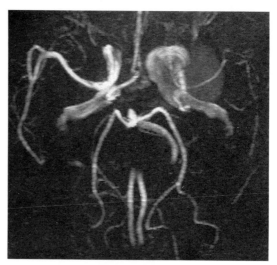

FIG. 40D. 3D TOF (FISP) 34/7/20°.

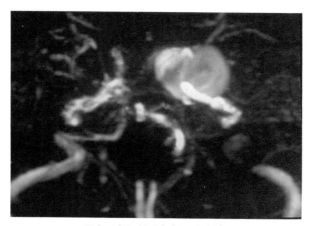

FIG. 40E. 3DPC 35/10/20°.

Clinical History

A 48-year-old female with progressive diplopia.

Findings

T1-weighted axial (Fig. 40A) and coronal (Fig. 40B) images demonstrate a heterogeneous mass lesion centered in the left cavernous carotid artery segment. The T2-weighted axial sequence (Fig. 40C) demonstrates flow-pulsation phase artifacts associated with the lesion. MR angiogram (Fig. 40D) depicts a giant aneurysm of the left cavernous carotid artery segment. Note the relative low signal intensity within the aneurysm lumen when compared with the phase contrast angiogram (Fig. 40E) done at the same sitting. However, the phase contrast angiogram utilized a relatively low velocity encoding (15 cm per second), accounting for poor visualization of the arterial structures when compared to the time-of-flight study and the better visualization of the slow intraaneurysmal flow. Intraarterial angiogram confirms the giant aneurysm (Fig. 40F).

Diagnosis

Giant cavernous carotid artery aneurysm.

Discussion

Aneurysms of the cavernous segment of the internal carotid artery will generally present with symptoms of mass effect rather than with subarachnoid hemorrhage. Ophthalmoplegia, headache, and even visual loss (due to impingement on the optic nerve) can develop. These lesions may rupture into the cavernous sinus to produce fistulization. MRA can miss small aneurysms of the cavernous segment; however, larger aneurysms, such as this, are easily depicted by MRA technique.

References

1. Olsen WL, Brant-Zawadzki MN, et al. Giant intracranial aneurysms: MR imaging. *Radiology* 1987;163:431–435.
2. Atlas SW, Grossman RI, et al. Partially thrombosed giant intracranial aneurysms: correlation of MR and pathologic findings. *Radiology* 1987;162:111–114.
3. Foss JS, Masaryk TJ, et al. Intracranial aneurysms: evaluation by MR angiography. *AJNR* 1990;11:449–456.
4. Sevich RJ, Tsuruda JS, et al. Three dimensional time-of-flight MR angiography in the evaluation of cerebral aneurysms. *J Comput Assist Tomogr* 1990;14(6):874–881.

Submitted by: Michael Brant-Zawadzki, M.D., F.A.C.R., Hoag Memorial Hospital, Newport Beach, California; Michael Brant-Zawadzki, M.D., F.A.C.R., Senior Editor.

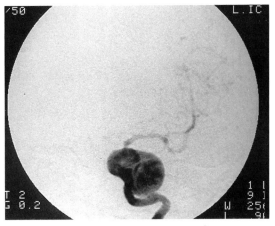

FIG. 40F. Intraarterial DSA LCA.

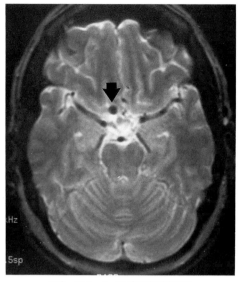

FIG. 41A. Axial SE 2500/90.

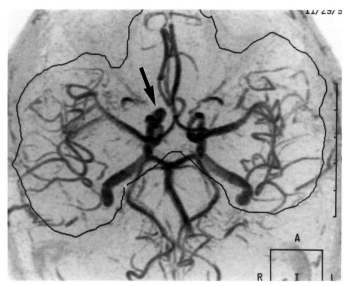

FIG. 41B. 3D TOF MOTSA 31/5.5/30° with ROI depiction.

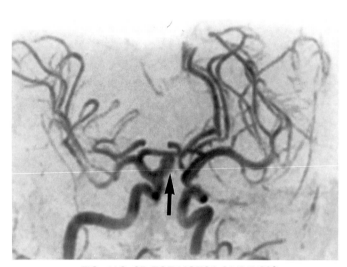

FIG. 41C. 3D TOF MOTSA 31/5.5/30°.

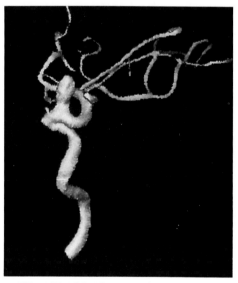

FIG. 41D. ISG Allegro surface rendering.

Clinical History

A 66-year-old female with headache.

Findings

T2-weighted axial image reveals a focal area of signal void in the region of the circle of Willis (Fig. 41A, *arrow*). The 3D MR angiography utilizing the multiple overlapping thin slab acquisition (MOTSA) technique verifies the presence of an aneurysm in the right supraclinoid carotid artery segment (Fig. 41B, *arrow*). Note that the freehand region of interest drawn around the vessels allows limited field of view reproduction of the intracranial vasculature, with rotation to best angle for depiction of the aneurysm (Fig. 41C, *arrow*). Also, surface rendering of the vessels is possible with workstation techniques (Fig. 41D). Conventional angiography demonstrates the aneurysm as well (Fig. 41E, *arrow*).

Diagnosis

Right periophthalamic internal carotid artery aneurysm.

Discussion

The MOTSA technique overcomes one of the disadvantages of 3D time-of-flight angiography. Namely, because the 3D slab volume is excited repeatedly, saturation effects can occur, limiting the resolution of vessels particularly deep in the slab. By subdividing the slab into smaller 3D segments, and adding them together, the saturation effects are minimized. The ability for freehand region of interest maximum intensity pixel reconstruction and surface rendering of the resulting vessel depiction enhances the display capabilities of MR angiography.

References

1. Blatter DD, Parker DL, et al. Cerebral MR angiography with multiple overlapping thin slab acquisition. Part I. Quantitative analysis of vessel visibility. *Radiology* 1991;179:805–811.
2. Blatter DD, Parker DL, et al. Cerebral MR angiography with multiple overlapping thin slab acquisition. Part II. Early clinical experience. *Radiology* 1992;183:379–389.
3. Lewin JS, Laub G. Intracranial MR angiography: a direct comparison of three time-of-flight techniques. *AJNR* 1992:12:1133–1139.

Submitted by: Evan Framm, M.D., Barrows Neurological Institute, St. Joseph's Hospital, Phoenix, Arizona; Michael Brant-Zawadzki, M.D., F.A.C.R., Senior Editor.

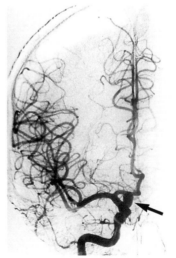

FIG. 41E. Intraarterial DSA, right carotid artery injection.

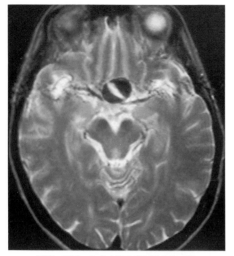

FIG. 42A. Axial SE 2800/22-90.

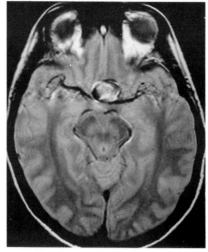

FIG. 42B. Axial SE 2800/22-90.

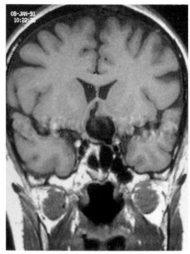

FIG. 42C. Coronal SE 600/15.

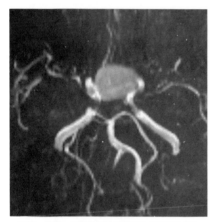

FIG. 42D. 3D TOF (FISP) 40/7/15°.

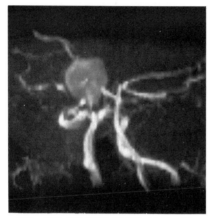

FIG. 42E. 3D TOF (FISP) 40/7/15°.

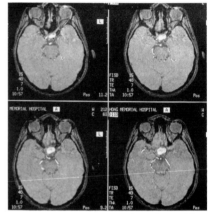

FIG. 42F. 3D TOF (FISP) 40/7/15°.

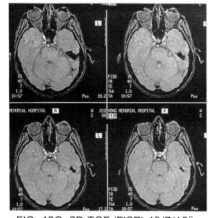

FIG. 42G. 3D TOF (FISP) 40/7/15°.

Clinical History

A 51-year-old female with visual difficulties.

Findings

Dual echo axial images (Figs. 42A and B) demonstrate a large lesion at the level of the anterior communicating artery, with heterogeneous signal and phase artifact emanating from the lesion. The T1-weighted coronal image (Fig. 42C) demonstrates the lesion to further advantage. Magnetic resonance angiography (MRA)-targeted maximum intensity pixel (MIP) images (Figs. 42D and E) depict a large high signal structure in the region of the anterior communicating artery. The MRA partition images (Figs. 42F and G) demonstrate this lesion; however, note that no definite aneurysm is seen of the cavernous carotid artery segment. Conventional angiogram (Figs. 42H and I) verifies the giant anterior communicating artery giant aneurysm, yet also depicts a small aneurysm off the subclinoid segment of the right internal carotid artery (*arrow*). This is not seen on the MRA partitions or on the subsequent projections.

Diagnosis

Giant anterior communicating artery aneurysm, with right cavernous carotid artery segment intradural aneurysm.

Discussion

This study again demonstrates the typical appearance of large aneurysms on conventional and time-of-flight angiographic sequences. As shown in Case 33, cavernous carotid segment aneurysms are very difficult to identify as such on MRA technique due to superimposition of the aneurysm with the tortuous morphology of the cavernous carotid artery segment. In addition, signal loss due to increased dephasing with turbulent flow and magnetic susceptibility effects from air–bone interfaces render this area difficult to image with MRA. Retrospective multiplanar reconstruction on the MRA data set with angle selection through the region of interest (Fig. 42J) reveals the right cavernous carotid artery aneurysm (*arrow*).

References

1. Olson WL, Brant-Zawadzki MN, et al. Giant intracranial aneurysms: MR imaging. *Radiology* 1987;163:431–435.
2. Atlas SW, Grossman RI, et al. Partially thrombosed giant intracranial aneurysms: correlation of MR and pathologic findings. *Radiology* 1987;162:111–114.
3. Ross JS, Masaryk TJ. Intracranial aneurysms: evaluation by MR angiography. *AJNR* 1990;11:449–456.
4. Sevick RJ, Tsuruda JS, et al. Three-dimensional time-of-flight MR angiography in the evaluation of cerebral aneurysms. *J Comput Assist Tomogr* 1990;14(6):874–881.

Submitted by: Michael Brant-Zawadzki, M.D., F.A.C.R., Hoag Memorial Hospital, Newport Beach, California; Michael Brant-Zawadzki, M.D., F.A.C.R., Senior Editor.

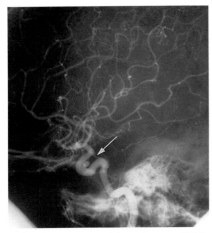

FIG. 42H. Intraarterial angiogram RCA.

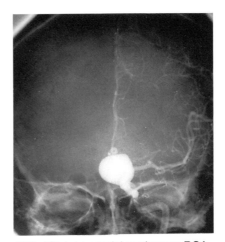

FIG. 42I. Intraarterial angiogram RCA.

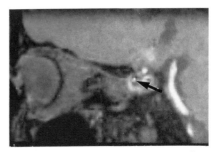

FIG. 42J. 3D TOF (FISP) 40/7/15°.

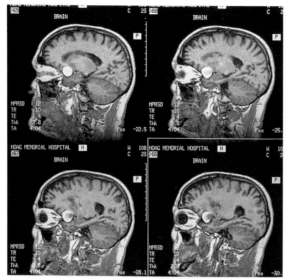

FIG. 43A. 3D MPRAGE 10/4/12°.

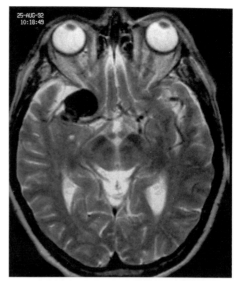

FIG. 43B. Axial Turbo SE 3500/93.

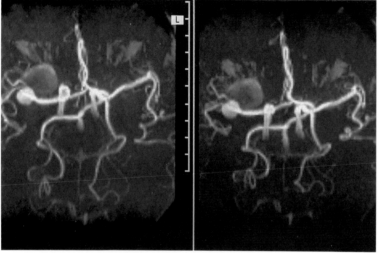

FIG. 43C. 3D TOF (FISP) 40/7/15°.

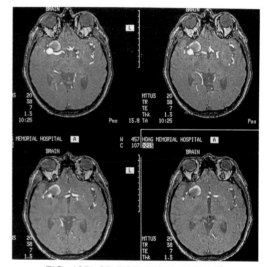

FIG. 43D. 3D TOF (FISP) 40/7/15°.

Clinical History

A 54-year-old male with a left-sided Bell's palsy.

Findings

T1-weighted sagittal and T2-weighted axial sequences (Figs. 43A and B) demonstrate a large mass in the region of the right middle cerebral artery trifurcation. However, this is an incidental finding, given the history of a left-sided Bell's palsy. The mass shows high signal intensity on the T1-weighted sequences and low signal intensity on the T2-weighted image. It is extraaxial, well circumscribed, and lobular in appearance. The MR angiogram (Fig. 43C) demonstrates the bilobular appearance of the abnormality at the middle cerebral artery trifurcation. The smaller, more posterolateral lobe contains high signal intensity consistent with flow. The more anterior component, with lower signal intensity, simply represents methemoglobin. The partitions (Fig. 43D) illustrate the differential signal in the flowing versus thrombosed component of the lesion.

Diagnosis

Giant aneurysm of the right middle cerebral artery trifurcation with partial thrombosis.

Discussion

Giant aneurysms tend to present with mass-like symptoms rather than subarachnoid hemorrhage. Detection of thrombus within the dome of a giant aneurysm is important as manipulation of the aneurysm at the time of surgery can lead to embolization from the thrombosed dome. Delineation of the neck of the aneurysm remains a key aspect of the approach to management. This is still best accomplished with intraarterial angiography (Fig. 43E).

Recently, the ability to acquire MR data in a three-dimensional format has aided the surgical approach to these patients. Figures 43F and G demonstrate the use of the original T1 data set (a 3D sequence) for synthesis of brain volume images in three dimensions. Superimposition of the MR angiographic data on the brain allows better orientation of the aneurysm to brain structure, thus optimizing surgical planning.

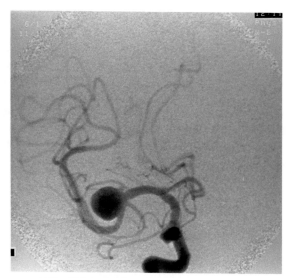

FIG. 43E. Intraarterial DSA RCA injection.

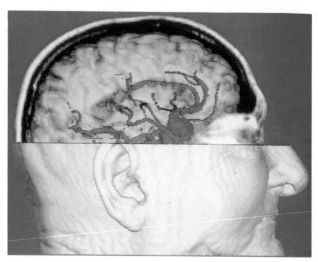

FIG. 43F. 3D surface reconstruction.

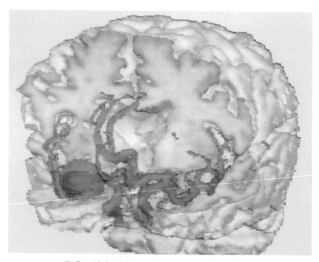

FIG. 43G. 3D surface reconstruction.

References

1. Ross JS, Masaryk TJ, et al. Intracranial aneurysms: evaluation by MR angiography. *AJNR* 1990;11:449–456.
2. Atlas SW, Grossman RI, et al. Partially thrombosed giant intracranial aneurysms: correlation of MR and pathologic findings. *Radiology* 1987;162:111–114.
3. Olsen WL, Brant-Zawadzki MN, et al. Giant intracranial aneurysms. *Radiology* 1987;163:431–435.
4. Cline HE, Lorensen WE, et al. 3D surface rendered MR images of the brain and its vasculature. *J Comput Assist Tomogr* 1991;15(2):344–351.
5. Hu X, Tan KK, et al. Three-dimensional magnetic resonance images of the brain: application to neurosurgical planning. *J Neurosurg* 1990;72:433–440.

Submitted by: Michael Brant-Zawadzki, M.D., F.A.C.R., Hoag Memorial Hospital, Newport Beach, California; Michael Brant-Zawadzki, M.D., F.A.C.R., Senior Editor.

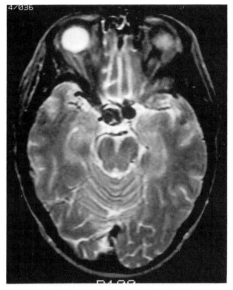
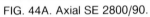

FIG. 44A. Axial SE 2800/90.

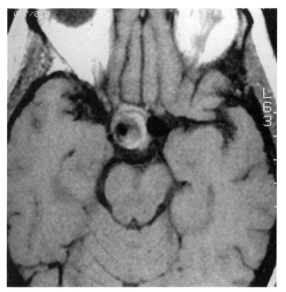

FIG. 44B. Axial SE 600/20.

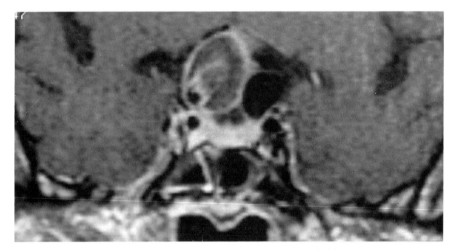

FIG. 44C. Postcontrast coronal SE 600/20.

Clinical History

A 64-year-old female with progressive visual loss.

Findings

The T2-weighted axial image demonstrates foci of signal void in the suprasellar region (Fig. 44A). The left supraclinoid carotid shows an aneurysmal structure with signal void and a more complex, heterogeneous signal mass is seen in relationship to the right supraclinoid artery (Fig. 44B). On the postcontrast coronal T1-weighted image (Fig. 44C) the right-sided mass is larger, and extends superiorly, compressing the optic chiasm.

Diagnosis

Bilateral supraclinoid carotid artery aneurysms with balloon occlusion on the right.

Discussion

The intraarterial angiograms demonstrate bilateral supraclinoid carotid artery aneurysms, the right associated with a stenotic segment of the supraclinoid carotid (Fig. 44D); the left associated with multiple lobulations, as well as a second aneurysm above the large dome projecting supramedially (Fig. 44E, *arrow*).

Anterioposterior post–balloon occlusion digital subtraction angiography (DSA) of the right-sided aneurysm (Fig. 44F) demonstrates almost complete closure of the aneurysm, as well as partial obstruction of the carotid lumen. The persistent thrombosed dome of the aneurysm can be inferred from the uplifted appearance of the right A-1 segment (*arrow*). Postocclusion MR image (Fig. 44G) shows the balloon as a focus of low signal intensity (*arrow*) within the dome of the right-sided giant aneurysm. Note the narrowed appearance of the carotid artery lumen (*arrowhead*). This study was obtained prior to the availability of MR angiography.

Subsequent follow-up MR angiogram (Fig. 44H) demonstrates increase in size of residual lumen in the treated right-sided aneurysm. The balloon has migrated up to the dome through the clot. The left-sided aneurysm remains, although its morphology is not shown to the advantage that intraarterial angiography allowed on the original study. Note that intravascular occlusion balloons show no signal on MR, thus may be mistaken for regions of flow void on routine or time-of-flight techniques.

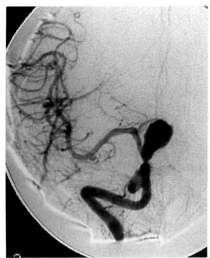

FIG. 44D. Intraarterial DSA RCA.

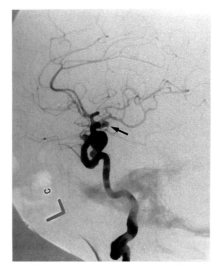

FIG. 44E. Intraarterial DSA LCA.

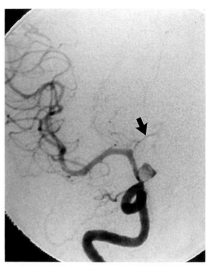

FIG. 44F. Intraarterial SDA RCA.

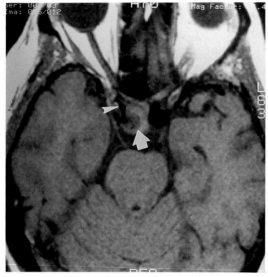

FIG. 44G. Axial SE 600/20.

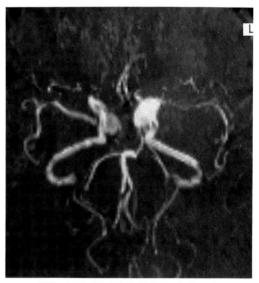

FIG. 44H. 3D TOF (FISP) 40/7/15°.

References

1. Kwan ES, Wolpert SM, et al. MR evaluation of the neurovascular lesions after endovascular occlusion with detachable balloons. *AJNR* 1988;9:523–531.

Submitted by: Michael Brant-Zawadzki, M.D., F.A.C.R., Hoag Memorial Hospital, Newport Beach, California; Michael Brant-Zawadzki, M.D., F.A.C.R., Senior Editor.

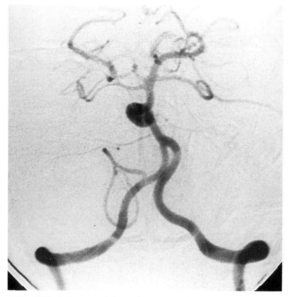

FIG. 45A. Intraarterial angiogram DSA AP oblique (aortic arch injection).

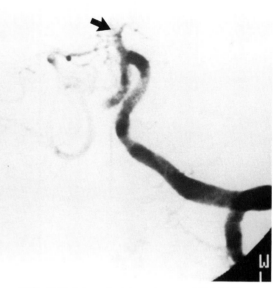

FIG. 45B. Intraarterial angiogram DSA LVA.

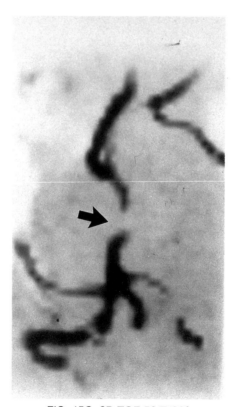

FIG. 45C. 3D TOF 50/7/20°.

Clinical History

A 30-year-old female with basilar artery aneurysm.

Findings

The preoperative intraarterial angiographic view of the midbasilar aneurysm is shown in Fig. 45A. After balloon detachment, a left vertebral intraarterial angiogram (Fig. 45B) demonstrates occlusion of the basilar artery above the level of balloon deployment (*arrow*) with retrograde filling of the distal contralateral vertebral artery. The post-therapy magnetic resonance angiogram (MRA) (Fig. 45C) obtained 5 days later demonstrates a filling defect in the midbasilar artery (*arrow*) with flow both above and below it. At 1 month post-therapy, the patient remains asymptomatic and follow-up MRA verifies persistent midbasilar artery occlusion with diminished flow in the vertebrals (Fig. 45D, *arrowheads*) and posterior cerebral (Fig. 45E, *arrowheads*) arteries.

Diagnosis

Midbasilar artery aneurysm with endovascular balloon occlusion.

Discussion

This patient was refused surgery by numerous neurosurgeons due to the high risk. The endovascular occlusion technique was the only option available and fortunately was successful in treating the aneurysm without neurologic complications. The MR angiogram after treatment verifies the persistent flow into the basilar above and below the level of occlusion. This case illustrates the advantage of MRA as a noninvasive follow-up examination.

References

1. Masaryk TJ, Modic MT, et al. Intracranial circulation: preliminary clinical results with three dimensional (volume) MR angiography. *Radiology* 1989;171:793–799.
2. Kwan ES, Wolpert SM, et al. MR evaluation of neurovascular lesions after endovascular occlusion with detachable balloons. *AJNR* 1988;9:523–531.
3. Sevick RJ, Tsuruda JS, et al. Three-dimensional time-of-flight MR angiography in the evaluation of cerebral aneurysms. *J Comput Assist Tomogr* 14(6):874–881.

Submitted by: Michael Brant-Zawadzki, M.D., F.A.C.R., Hoag Memorial Hospital, Newport Beach, California; Michael Brant-Zawadzki, M.D., F.A.C.R., Senior Editor.

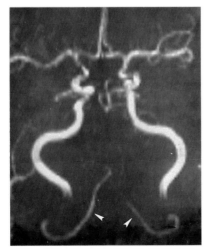

FIG. 45D. 3D TOF (FISP) 40/7/15°.

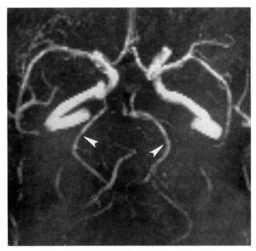

FIG. 45E. 3D TOF (FISP) 40/7/15°.

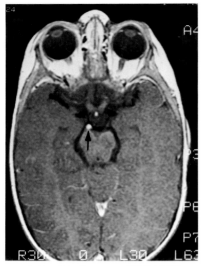

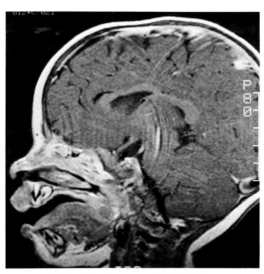

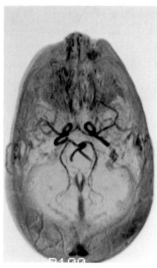

FIG. 46A. Contrast SE 500/20.

FIG. 46B. Contrast SE 500/20.

FIG. 46C. 3D TOF MRA 2D collapsed.

Clinical History

A 7-month-old with right third cranial nerve palsy (oculomotor).

Findings

Axial T1-weighted image with contrast (Fig. 46A) shows a nodular enhancing mass uplifting the right posterior cerebral artery (PCA). Sagittal T1-weighted image better demonstrates the enhancing right third nerve (Fig. 46B). The 3D time-of-flight (TOF) magnetic resonance angiography (MRA) shows no evidence for aneurysm of the PCA (Fig. 46C).

Diagnosis

Oculomotor nerve palsy without evidence for aneurysm.

Discussion

The differential diagnosis for third cranial nerve palsy (1) includes ischemic microvascular disease, brain stem lesions, aneurysm of the circle of Willis or cavernous sinus, and lesions in the orbital apex. In adults the most common cause is ischemia associated with diabetes mellitus. In children the most common cause for oculomotor nerve deficit is congenital, then trauma or infection (2). Aneurysm is unusual. Normally, the third cranial nerve does not enhance. Although not biopsied, the enhancement associated with the third cranial nerve in this case is most likely secondary to an inflammatory process or a tumor such as papillary meningioma (3).

References

1. Kwan ESK, Laucella M, Hedges TR, Wolpert SM. A cliniconeuroradiologic approach to third cranial nerve palsies. *AJNR* 1987;8:459–468.
2. Miller NR. Solitary oculomotor nerve palsy in childhood. *Am J Ophthalmol* 1977;83:106–111.
3. Piatt JH, Campbell GA, Oakes WJ. Papillary meningioma involving the oculomotor nerve in an infant. *J Neurosurg* 1986;64:808–812.

Submitted by: Orest B. Boyko, M.D., Ph.D., Duke University Medical Center, Durham, North Carolina; Michael Brant-Zawadzki, M.D., F.A.C.R., Senior Editor.

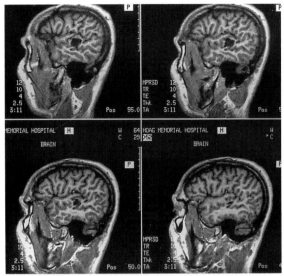

FIG. 47A. 3D sagittal (MP RAGE) 10/4/12°.

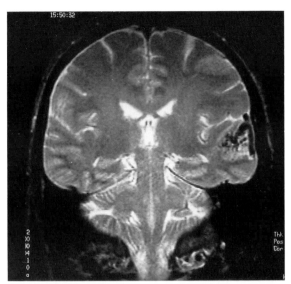

FIG. 47B. Coronal SE 2800/90.

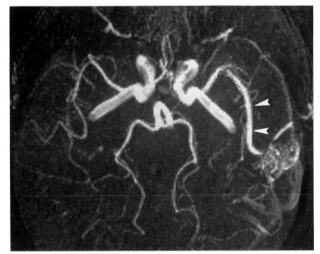

FIG. 47C. 3D TOF (FISP) 40/7/15°.

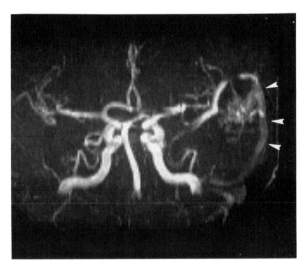

FIG. 47D. 3D TOF (FISP) 40/7/15°.

Clinical History

A 39-year-old male with uncontrollable seizures and transient aphasia.

Findings

T1-weighted sagittal images (Fig. 47A) show serpentine structures within the left temporal lobe. The coronal T2-weighted image (Fig. 47B) suggests a large cortical draining vein from the nidus of the abnormality. The MR angiographic views show the malformation in the basal and brow-up rotations (Figs. 47C and D, respectively). A single large feeding branch from the middle cerebral artery system is seen leading to the nidus (Fig. 47C, *arrowheads*); the venous drainage on the cortical surface (Fig. 47D, *arrowheads*) of the temporal lobe is best demonstrated on the brow-up view.

The intraarterial angiogram (Fig. 47E) verifies the malformation, and also shows the venous drainage to better advantage with the vein of Labbé (*arrow*) and Trolard (*curved arrow*) nicely depicted. Postsurgical views (Fig. 47F) demonstrate the preservation of the feeding branch (*arrow*), as well as the distal branch from the feeder, with complete obliteration of the malformation.

Diagnosis

Left temporal lobe arteriovenous malformation (AVM).

Discussion

Small AVMs with rapid shunts can easily be depicted even with conventional spin-echo MR images. MR angiographic views can help depict the routes of feeding and draining vessels to better advantage. Although not utilized in this case, selective presaturation can aid in the determination of specific feeding vessels as that portion of the AVM supplied by the presaturated vessel would have a marked reduction in signal. Again, intraarterial angiographic studies are necessary for surgical planning in these patients, due to its superior spatial and temporal resolution.

References

1. Le Blanc R, Levesque M, et al. Magnetic resonance imaging of arteriovenous malformations. *Neurosurgery* 1987;21:15–20.
2. Edelman R, Wentz KU, et al. Intracerebral arteriovenous malformations: evaluation with selective MR angiography and venography. *Radiology* 1989;173:831–837.
3. Nassel F, Weymuller H, et al. Comparison of magnetic resonance angiography, magnetic resonance imaging and conventional angiography in cerebral arteriovenous malformation. *Neuroradiology* 1991;33:55–61.

Submitted by: Michael Brant-Zawadzki, M.D., F.A.C.R., Hoag Memorial Hospital, Newport Beach, California; Michael Brant-Zawadzki, M.D., F.A.C.R., Senior Editor.

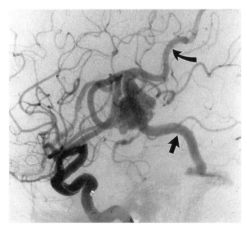

FIG. 47E. Intraarterial DSA LCA.

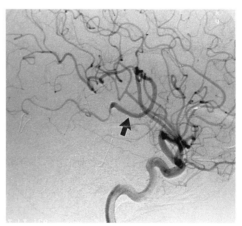

FIG. 47F. Intraarterial DSA LCA.

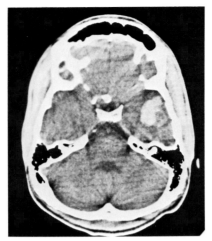

FIG. 48A. Non-contrast CT.

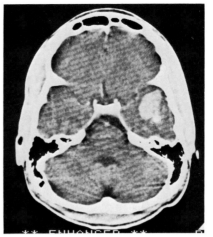

FIG. 48B. Contrast CT.

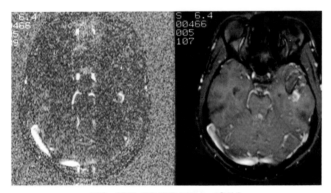

FIG. 48C. 2D PC MRA, 49/11.

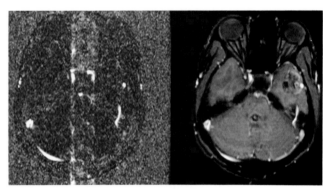

FIG. 48D. 2D PC MRA, 49/11.

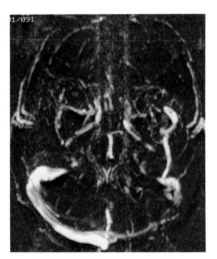

FIG. 48E. 2D PC MRA, 45/12.

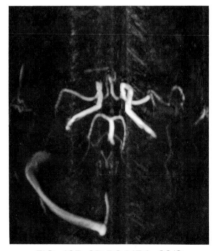

FIG. 48F. 3D PC MRA, 36/8.

Clinical History

A 16-year-old male with acute seizure.

Findings

Noncontrast CT scan shows an acute left temporal lobe hematoma (Fig. 48A) with a focal area of contrast enhancement (Fig. 48B). This region shows hyperintense signal, indicating flow-related enhancement (FRE), on the phase (Fig. 48C, *left*) and the magnitude (Fig. 48C, *right*) images on 2D phase contrast (PC) magnetic resonance angiography (MRA) using a velocity encoding of 80 cm/sec. More posteriorly a draining vein into the left transverse sinus can be seen (Fig. 48D). The 2D collapsed reprojection image demonstrates the prominent draining vein (Fig. 48E) at a velocity encoding of 20 cm/sec. Note on a 3D PC MRA with velocity encoding of 80 cm/sec the poor visualization of the draining vein as well as the transverse sinus due to saturation effects (Fig. 48F).

Diagnosis

Hemorrhage from arteriovenous malformation (AVM) left temporal lobe.

Discussion

Conventional angiogram showed a small arteriovenous nidus supplied by an anterior temporal branch of the left middle cerebral artery. In this case the small nidus was difficult to see on the MRA. The draining vein is well shown by MRA and the 2D PC MRA gives excellent subtraction on the phase and speed images of the complex signal intensities of the blood clot, leaving hyperintense signal of only flowing blood.

References

1. Edelman RR, Wentz KU, Mattle HP, et al. Intracerebral arteriovenous malformation: evaluation with selective MR angiography and venography. *Radiology* 1989;173:831–837.
2. Nassel F, Weymuller H, Huber P. Comparison of magnetic resonance angiography, magnetic resonance imaging and conventional angiography in cerebral arteriovenous malformation. *Neuroradiology* 1991;33:56–61.

Submitted by: Orest B. Boyko, M.D., Ph.D., Duke University Medical Center, Durham, North Carolina; Michael Brant-Zawadzki, M.D., F.A.C.R., Senior Editor.

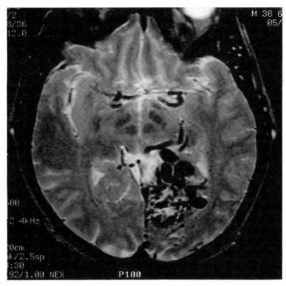

FIG. 49A. Axial SE 2500/91.

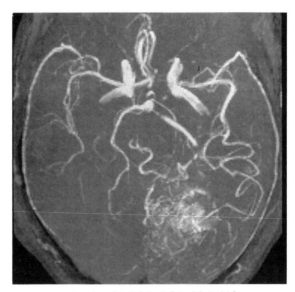

FIG. 49B. 3D TOF (FISP) 30/7/20°.

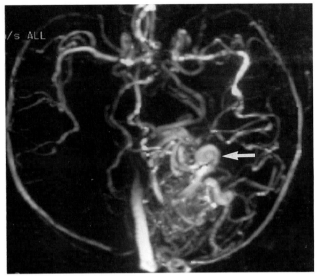

FIG. 49C. PC MRA 34/9/20°.

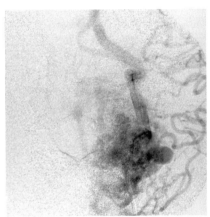

FIG. 49D. Intraarterial angiogram DSA LCA.

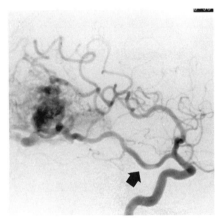

FIG. 49E. Intraarterial angiogram DSA LCA.

Clinical History

A 38-year-old male with seizures.

115

Findings

The T2-weighted spin-echo image (Fig. 49A) demonstrates a large nidus of serpentine structures in the left calcarine region. Several of the prominent signal void foci suggest variceal dilatation or aneurysm formation. The MRA base view (Fig. 49B) shows the nidus of the malformation, but fails to reveal any discrete variceal structures. The phase contrast angiogram base view (Fig. 49C) was performed with a velocity encoding of 40 cm/sec (in all directions). This does depict the most prominent of the variceal-like outpouchings in the anterolateral aspect of the malformation (*arrow*). The base view from the intraarterial angiogram (Fig. 49D) shows the corresponding varix to good advantage, and depicts the major feeding vessel, which is posterior cerebral artery (Fig. 49D). The posterior middle cerebral artery branches contribute to the malformation as well.

Diagnosis

Left occipital lobe arteriovenous malformation, with variceal enlargement of the draining veins.

Discussion

This set of figures demonstrates some differences between the time-of-flight technique and the phase contrast technique. First of all, note the improved background suppression with phase contrast angiography. Note also that the ability to depict more slowly flowing structures such as veins is more readily available with the manipulation of velocity encoding during phase contrast angiography. The detection of varices is important, as their presence raises the risk for hemorrhage from arteriovenous malformation, and usually implies restriction of venous outflow from the malformation. It is clear, however, that the intraarterial angiogram is still the most definitive technique for evaluating arteriovenous malformations. The exact delineation of feeding vessels, particularly if intervention through endovascular or surgical routes is anticipated, requires conventional angiography. Note, for instance, the questionable appearance of the posterior cerebral artery feeding vessel on both the time-of-flight and the phase contrast angiograms as compared with the definitive appearance of the feeder on the intraarterial DSA study (Fig. 49E, *arrow*). Nevertheless, identifying the full nidus of the malformation, and following it through therapy makes magnetic resonance a useful modality in the diagnostic armamentarium.

References

1. Huston J III, Rufenacht DA, et al. Intracranial aneurysms and vascular malformations: comparison of time-of-flight and phase contrast angiography. *Radiology* 1991;181:721–730.
2. Leblanc R, Levesque M, et al. Magnetic resonance imaging of cerebral arteriovenous malformations. *Neurosurgery* 1987;21:15–20.
3. Atlas SW. Intracranial vascular malformations and aneurysms. In: Atlas SW, ed. *Magnetic resonance imaging of the brain and spine.* New York: Raven Press, 1991;379–410.

Submitted by: Michael Brant-Zawadzki, M.D., F.A.C.R., Hoag Memorial Hospital, Newport Beach, California; Michael Brant-Zawadzki, M.D., F.A.C.R., Senior Editor.

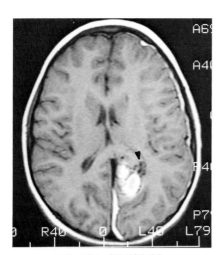

FIG. 50A. SE 500/20.

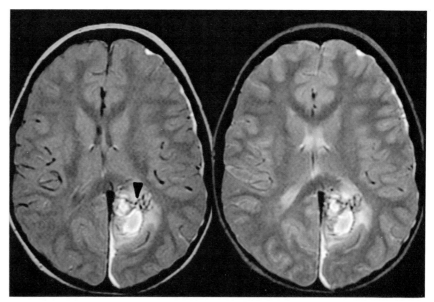

FIG. 50B. SE 2000/80.

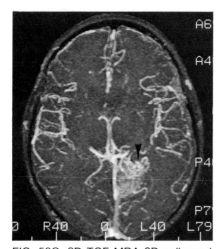

FIG. 50C. 2D TOF MRA 2D collapsed post-processed (GRE 45/8/60).

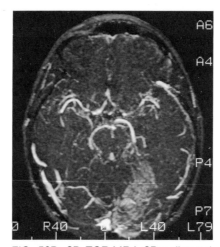

FIG. 50D. 2D TOF MRA 2D collapsed post-processed (GRE 45/8/60).

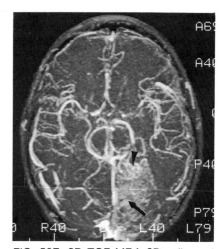

FIG. 50E. 2D TOF MRA 2D collapsed (GRE 45/8/60).

Clinical History

An 8-year-old male with left-sided headache and seizure.

Findings

T1-weighted MR image 2 days after admission (Fig. 50A) demonstrates a left occipital lobe hyperintense hematoma with medial occipital lobe and frontotemporal lobe subdural. Posterior to the left splenium of the corpus callosum are multiple flow voids (Fig. 50A, *arrowhead*). T2-weighted image (Fig. 50B) shows hyperintense methemoglobin of the hematoma, edema, and hypointense flow voids posterior and to the left of the splenium (Fig. 50B, *arrowhead*). The 2D time-of-flight (TOF) magnetic resonance angiography (MRA) 2D collapsed image shows hyperintense left occipital lobe thrombus (Fig. 50C, *arrow*), mimicking flow-related enhancement (FRE) and actual FRE of the vascular malformation nidus (Fig. 50C, *arrowhead*). Further postprocessing using selective 2D collapsed images at the level of the posterior cerebral arteries (Fig. 50D) highlights the clot and at the level of the internal cerebral veins highlights the nidus (Fig. 50E, *arrowhead*). Intraarterial DSA (F) depicts the vascular malformation as well.

Diagnosis

Methemoglobin hematoma secondary to hemorrhage from a left occipital lobe arteriovenous malformation (AVM).

Discussion

MR imaging can be superior to MRA and conventional angiography in demonstrating AVMs (1,2). As this case illustrates hyperintense signal on gradient echo pulse sequences used in MRA acquisitions can result from the short T1 of methemoglobin mimicking FRE, which is less intense than FRE in the actual malformation.

References

1. Nassel F, Wegmuller H, Huber P. Comparison of magnetic resonance angiography, magnetic resonance imaging and conventional angiography in cerebral arteriovenous malformation. *Neuroradiology* 1991;33:56–61.
2. Edelman RR, Wentz KU, Mattle HP, et al. Intracerebral arteriovenous malformations: evaluation with selective MR angiography and venography. *Radiology* 1989;173:831–837.
3. Yousem DM, Balakrishnan J, Debrun GM, et al. Hyperintense thrombus on GRASS MR images: potential pitfall in flow evaluation. *AJNR* 1990;11:51–58.

Submitted by: Orest B. Boyko, M.D., Ph.D., Duke University Medical Center, Durham, North Carolina; Michael Brant-Zawadzki, M.D., F.A.C.R., Senior Editor.

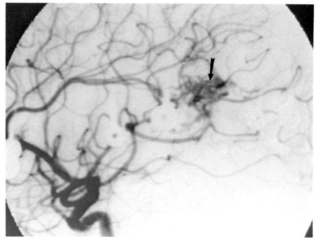

FIG. 50F. Intracranial DSA LCA.

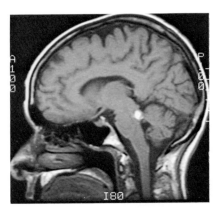

FIG. 51A. SE 500/20.

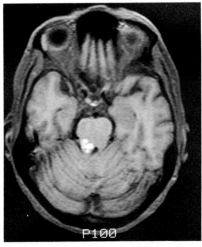

FIG. 51B. SE 500/20.

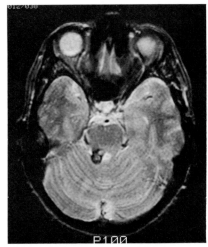

FIG. 51C. SE 2000/80.

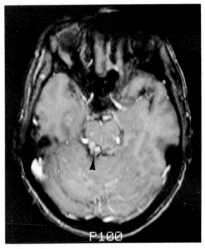

FIG. 51D. 2D PC MRA (24/10/45°).
Magnitude image.

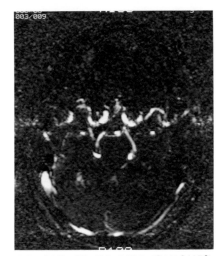

FIG. 51E. 2D PC MRA (24/10/45°).
Speed image.

Clinical History

A 56-year-old female presents with right-hand weakness and left spinothalamic tract findings.

Findings

Sagittal T1-weighted image (Fig. 51A) demonstrates a hyperintense lesion in the dorsal midbrain, anterior to the colliculi. Axial T1-weighted image with frequency selective fat suppression pulse sequence (Fig. 51B) demonstrates no saturation of the hyperintense signal, indicating that lipid does not account for the T1 shortening. Note the suppression of orbital fat signal. T2-weighted spin-echo (Fig. 51C) images shows a hypointense rim indicative of hemosiderin.

The 2D phase contrast (PC) magnetic resonance angiography (MRA) shows the area of hyperintense methemoglobin remains hyperintense on the magnitude image (Fig. 51D, *arrowhead*), mimicking flow. Speed image documents that no signal (thus no flow) is present in the lesion (Fig. 51E) at a velocity encoding (VENC) of 20 cm/sec. Conventional angiogram was negative.

Diagnosis

Cavernous malformation (angioma) of the brain stem.

Discussion

Vascular malformations can be divided into four categories: arteriovenous malformation (AVM), venous malformation, capillary telangiectasia, and cavernous malformation (the latter two being occult on conventional angiograms). Pathologically cavernous angiomas are formed of thin-walled vascular spaces that can be thrombosed, but with no intervening brain tissue and no arterialized veins. Hemosiderin-laden macrophages are present histologically, accounting for the areas of T2 hypointense signal. T2 signal intensity centrally tends to be mixed.

A familial incidence for cavernous malformations has been reported.

The maximum pixel intensity algorithm that generates vessel morphology can mistake high signal from blood for vessels on TOF MRA. In this case 2D PC MRA helped distinguish hyperintense signal of methemoglobin from flow-related enhancement. As with conventional angiography, MRA does not show flow in these lesions.

References

1. Rigamonti D, Drayer BP, Johnson PC, et al. The MRI appearance of cavernous malformations (angiomas). *J Neurosurg* 1987;67:518–524.
2. Zimmerman RS, Spetzler RF, Lee KS, et al. Cavernous malformation of the brain stem. *J Neurosurg* 1991;75:32–39.

Submitted by: Orest B. Boyko, M.D., Ph.D., Duke University Medical Center, Durham, North Carolina; Michael Brant-Zawadzki, M.D., F.A.C.R., Senior Editor.

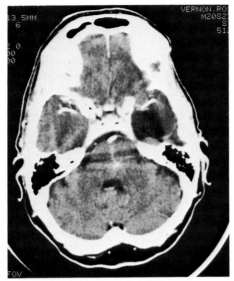

FIG. 52A. Contrast CT scan.

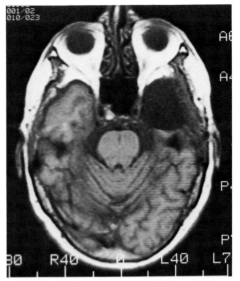

FIG. 52B. SE 500/20.

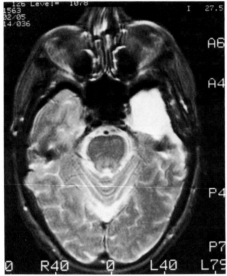

FIG. 52C. SE 2800/80.

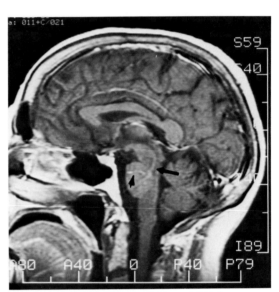

FIG. 52D. Contrast T1-weighted

Clinical History

A 66-year-old female with previous left temporal lobe resection.

Findings

Contrast CT scan shows left temporal lobe resection with radiating spoke wheel and tubular enhancement within the pons (Fig. 52A). Axial T1-weighted image shows the ventral tubular structure (Fig. 52B), which is not visualized on T2-weighted image (Fig. 52C).

Contrast-enhanced sagittal T1-weighted image shows pontine enhancement ventral and superior (Fig. 52D, *arrows*). Note the presence of contrast and hyperintense signal in venous structures such as the internal cerebral vein.

Diagnosis

Pontine venous angioma.

Discussion

Venous angiomas are considered a developmental anomaly. Their clinical significance is controversial, with supratentorial lesions having been associated with seizure or headache and posterior fossa locations with headache, vertigo, dizziness, tinnitus, nystagmus, or ataxia. Hemorrhage or venous infarct is rare. As this case illustrates, venous angiomas can be obscured on spin-echo imaging because of partial volume averaging and slow velocities masking time-of-flight effects (1). Contrast MR can improve the detection of venous angiomas (32% increase in visualization shown in one series) (2). The slow venous flow in venous angiomas accounts for the pooling of T1 shortening and apparent enhancement and must be distinguished from enhancement due to pathologic processes such as multiple sclerosis or tumor.

References

1. Wilms G, Marchal G, Van Hecke P, et al. Cerebral venous angiomas. MR imaging at 1.5 tesla. *Neuroradiology* 1990;32:81–85.
2. Wilms G, Demaerel P, Marchal G, et al. Gadolinium-enhanced MR imaging of cerebral venous angiomas with emphasis on their drainage. *J Comput Assist Tomogr* 1991;15:199–206.

Submitted by: Orest B. Boyko, M.D., Ph.D., Duke University Medical Center, Durham, North Carolina; Michael Brant-Zawadzki, M.D., F.A.C.R., Senior Editor.

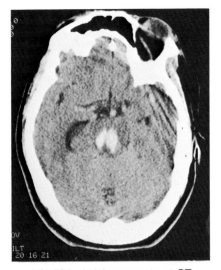

FIG. 53A. Axial non-contrast CT.

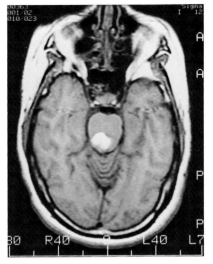

FIG. 53B. SE 500/20.

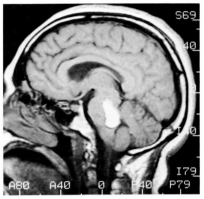

FIG. 53C. SE 500/20.

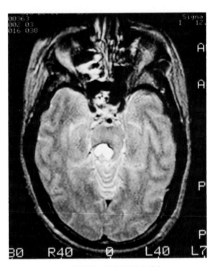

FIG. 53D. SE 2000/80.

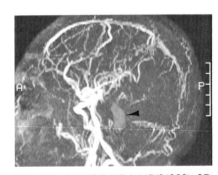

FIG. 53E. 2D TOF MRA (45/9/60°). 3D reprojections.

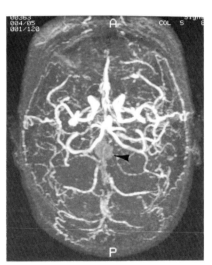

FIG. 53F. 2D TOF MRA (45/9/60°). 2D collapsed reprojection.

Clinical History

A 49-year-old female presents with acute headache and facial weakness.

Findings

Non-contrast CT scan shows an acute hyperdense midbrain hemorrhage (Fig. 53A). T1-weighted MR images 3 weeks later (Figs. 53B and C) show the presence of methemoglobin (bright signal intensity or T1 shortening). T2-weighted MR image confirms high signal intensity of dilute-free methemoglobin with a partial peripheral hemosiderin rim of hypointense signal (T2 shortening).

The 2D time-of-flight (TOF) magnetic resonance angiography (MRA) demonstrates the expected low signal intensity of stationary protons of the brain but bright signal intensity of the stationary protons of the thrombus is seen. This mimics flow-related enhancement (FRE) (Figs. 53E and F, *arrowhead*). Conventional angiography demonstrated no arteriovenous malformation.

Diagnosis

Midbrain hematoma from occult cerebrovascular malformation (OCVM).

Discussion

The 2D TOF MRA technique uses a gradient recalled echo pulse sequence. Flowing spins (blood) will have hyperintense signal due to the presence of (a) entry-slice phenomenon on each sequential slice acquisition, (b) the use of flow compensation gradients, and (c) the lack of 90° and 180° slice-selective pulses, which would normally minimize time-of-flight effects. All these factors account for the lack of flow void phenomenon on gradient recalled echo images.

A potential pitfall in interpretation of 2D TOF MRA is the fact that stationary protons in blood products have a short T1 (as in this case due to methemoglobin) and can be hyperintense on gradient recalled echoes images (1) mimicking FRE. Flip angle, TR, and TE influence the contribution of signal intensity from the T1, T2, and spin density characteristics of the stationary protons. A 2D TOF MRA pulse sequence, having a flip angle of 60° and a short TE of 9 msec, has T1-weighting and will be sensitive to paramagnetic material such as methemoglobin. Routine spin-echo imaging can be useful in the diagnosis and follow-up of OCVM. Normal evolution of signal intensity changes by red blood cells or new areas of bleeding can be shown (2).

References

1. Yousem DM, Balakrishnan J, Debrun GM, et al. Hyperintense thrombus on GRASS MR images: potential pitfall in flow evaluation. *AJNR* 1990;11:51–58.
2. Sigal R, Krief O, Houtteville JP, et al. Occult cerebrovascular malformations: follow-up with MR imaging. *Radiology* 1990;176:815–819.

Submitted by: Orest B. Boyko, M.D., Ph.D., Duke University Medical Center, Durham, North Carolina; Michael Brant-Zawadzki, M.D., F.A.C.R., Senior Editor.

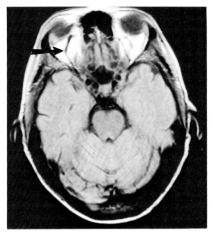

FIG. 54A. SE 2250/20.

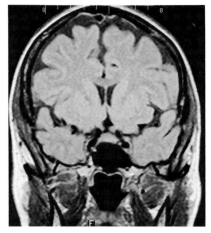

FIG. 54B. SE 2100/20.

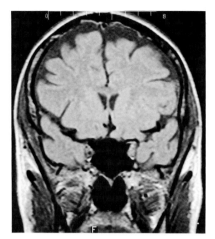

FIG. 54C. SE 2100/20.

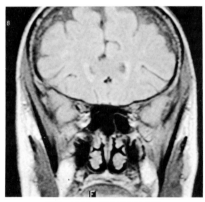

FIG. 54D. SE 2100/20.

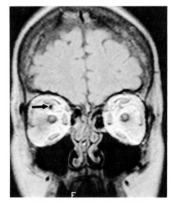

FIG. 54E. SE 2100/20.

126

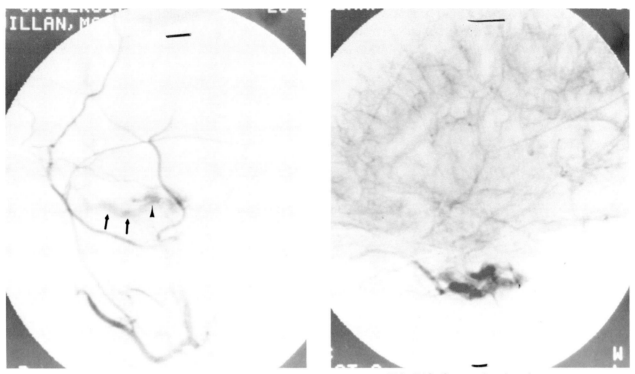

FIG. 54F. Conventional angiogram.

FIG. 54G. Conventional angiogram.

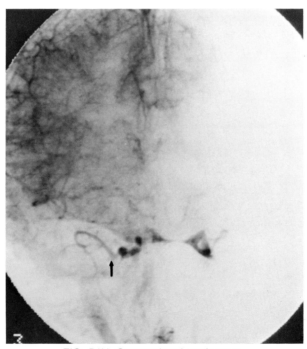

FIG. 54H. Conventional angiogram.

Clinical History

A 54-year-old female with double vision and an injected, chemotic right eye.

Findings

Axial proton density image reveals dilated right superior ophthalmic vein (SOV) with a more pronounced flow void than the left SOV (Fig. 54A, *arrow*). Coronal proton density image (Fig. 54B) shows dilatation of the right cavernous internal carotid artery (ICA), suggesting atherosclerotic change with no asymmetry to the size of the right cavernous sinus. Further images through the orbit (Figs. 54C–E) confirm dilated right SOV (Figs. 54C–E, *arrow*) with a more pronounced flow void.

Conventional selective right external carotid artery (ECA) lateral angiogram shows in the early arterial phase dense filling of the right cavernous sinus (Fig. 54F, *arrowhead*) and venous drainage through a dilated SOV (Fig. 54F, *arrows*). Late lateral arterial phase of a right common carotid artery (CCA) injection (Fig. 54G) shows the early filling of the cavernous sinus and SOV. Note the SOV on anteroposterior (AP) projection (Fig. 54H, *arrow*).

Diagnosis

Right cavernous sinus dural arteriovenous malformation (AVM).

Discussion

Cavernous sinus "fistulas" can result from arteriovenous malformations of the dura around the cavernous sinus fed by meningeal branches of the ECA, or by direct fistula communication between the ICA itself and the cavernous sinus (due to trauma, or aneurysmal rupture).

Most ECA-cavernous sinus communications are based on the preexistence of an arteriovenous malformation connection between the meningeal arterial branches and the dural veins in the cavernous sinus. Spontaneous opening of such anastomoses can occur because of hypertension, atherosclerosis, or trauma.

The clinical findings of an orbital bruit, chemosis, and pulsating exophthalmus are due to transmission of arterial pressure to the cavernous sinus with draining into a dilated SOV.

Decreased MR signal intensity in the involved cavernous sinus has been reported (2) with dural AVM and is reported to be representative of a high-velocity signal loss due to the rapid flow arteriovenous shunt.

References

1. Peters FLM, Kroger R. Dural and direct cavernous sinus fistulas. *AJR* 1979;132:599–606.
2. Hirabuki N, Miura T, Harada K, et al. MR imaging of dural arteriovenous malformations with ocular signs. *Neuroradiology* 1988;30:390–394.

Submitted by: Orest B. Boyko, M.D., Ph.D., Duke University Medical Center, Durham, North Carolina; Michael Brant-Zawadzki, M.D., F.A.C.R., Senior Editor.

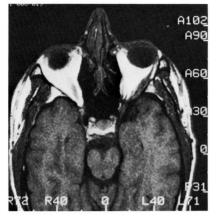

FIG. 55A. SE 500/20.

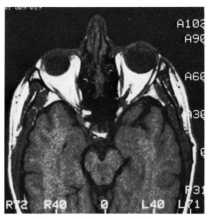

FIG. 55B. SE 500/20.

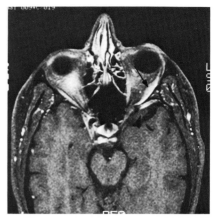

FIG. 55C. SE 500/20 postcontrast with frequency selective fat saturation.

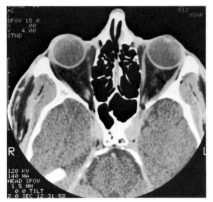

FIG. 55D. Axial orbital CT with contrast.

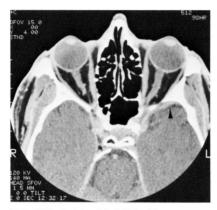

FIG. 55E. Axial orbital CT with contrast.

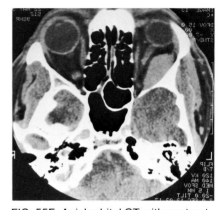

FIG. 55F. Axial orbital CT with contrast, post Valsalva.

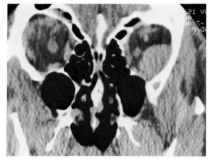

FIG. 55G. Coronal orbital CT with contrast in head hanging position.

Clinical History

A 49-year-old male complaining of left orbital positional exophthalmos.

Findings

T1-weighted orbital MR images (Figs. 55A and B) show no retrobulbar mass but a thickened medial border of the left lateral rectus muscle (LRM). T1-weighted image with contrast and fat suppression saturation pulse (Fig. 55C) shows normal enhancement of the extraocular muscles. There is an enhancing outpouching of the medial border of the left LRM (Fig. 55C, *arrow*) and a prominent left sphenoparietal venous sinus (Fig. 55C, *arrowhead*). CT scan also shows the left LRM medial border prominence (Fig. 55D, *arrow*) with prominent left sphenoparietal venous sinus (Fig. 55E, *arrowhead*). Axial CT scan with the patient performing a Valsalva maneuver (Fig. 55F) or coronal CT scan in a hanging head position (Fig. 55G) shows an enhancing retrobulbar mass that displaces the optic nerve medially.

Diagnosis

Left orbital varix.

Discussion

Causes for intermittent exophthalmos include orbital varix, hemangioma or lymphangioma associated with periodic congestion, and lacrimal gland hyperplasia. Primary orbital varices are congenital or traumatic and secondary varices are due to intracranial or orbital arteriovenous malformation or carotid-cavernous fistula. Associated exophthalmos can be elicited by coughing, straining, Valsalva, jugular vein compression, or leaning forward. MR reports have been sporadic (1, 2) but this case illustrates that the medial left LRM enhancement was actually contrast pooling in the collapsed varix. This is comparable to the pooling of contrast in the cavernous sinus. The prominent left sphenoparietal sinus was secondary to increased venous drainage from the orbital varix.

References

1. Osborn RE, DeWitt JD, Lester PD, et al. Magnetic resonance imaging of an orbital varix with CT and ultrasound correlation. *Comput Radiol* 1986;10:155–159.
2. Wildenhain PM, Lehar SC, Dastur KJ, et al. Orbital varix: color flow imaging correlated with CT and MR studies. *J Comput Assist Tomogr* 1991;15:171–173.

Submitted by: Orest B. Boyko, M.D., Ph.D., Duke University Medical Center, Durham, North Carolina; Michael Brant-Zawadzki, M.D., F.A.C.R., Senior Editor.

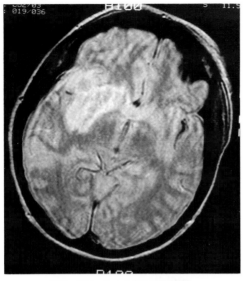

FIG. 56A. Axial SE 2800/30.

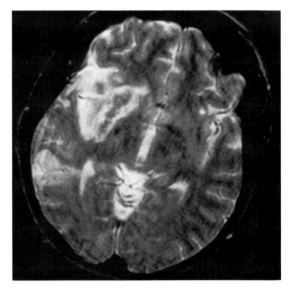

FIG. 56B. Axial SE 2800/90.

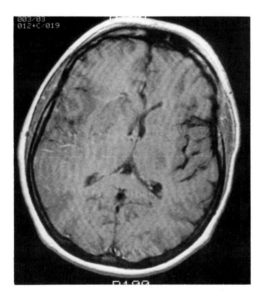

FIG. 56C. Axial SE postcontrast 800/20.

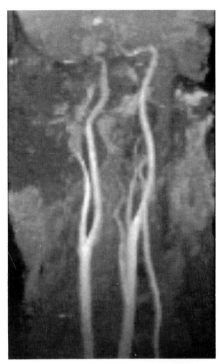

FIG. 56D. 3D TOF (FISP) 40/7/30°.

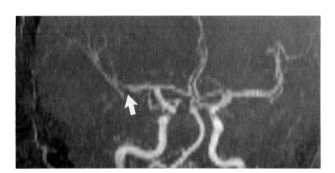

FIG. 56E. 3D TOF (FISP) 40/7/20°.

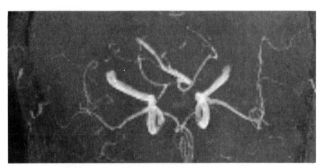

FIG. 56F. 3D TOF (FISP) 40/7/20°.

Clinical History

A 44-year-old female with sudden onset of left hemiparesis following hysterectomy for carcinoma of the cervix.

Findings

The MRI study demonstrates an infarct in the right anterior temporal and basal ganglia distribution of the middle cerebral artery (Figs. 56A and B). The postcontrast T1-weighted axial image (Fig. 56C) demonstrates asymmetric enhancement of the middle cerebral artery branches. Magnetic resonance angiographic (MRA) study clears the carotids as a source of embolus (Fig. 56D). The intracranial 3D time-of-flight study (Fig. 56E) demonstrates asymmetry in the horizontal portion of the middle cerebral artery segment with a focal flow defect in the distal M-1 segment (*arrow*). Also, the right middle cerebral artery branches are less detailed, particularly on the base view (Fig. 56F).

Diagnosis

Embolic infarction of right middle cerebral artery.

Discussion

This study demonstrates the value of MR angiography in the acute infarct patient. The dual echo sequences demonstrate infarction with suggestion of hemorrhagic conversion particularly in the basal ganglia. This is seen on the second echo image, as well as on partitions from the MR angiogram that accentuate the magnetic susceptibility effects of blood (Fig. 56G). Fearing a hypercoagulable state in this posthysterectomy patient, the clinicians chose not to do intraarterial angiography but opted for the MR angiogram instead, which proved the carotids to be free of occlusive disease. The embolic nature of the infarction is well demonstrated on MRA with the typical site of embolus lodging at the middle cerebral artery trifurcation. Also, hemorrhagic conversion is a common feature of embolic infarction.

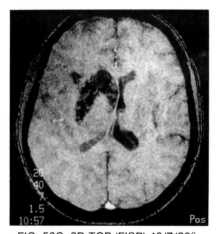

FIG. 56G. 3D TOP (FISP) 40/7/20°.

References

1. Warach S, Li W, et al. Acute cerebral ischemia: evaluation with dynamic contrast-enhanced MR imaging and MR angiography. *Radiology* 1992;182:41–47.
2. Masary, TJ, Modic MT, et al. Intracranial circulation: preliminary clinical results with three-dimensional (volume) MR angiography. *Radiology* 1989;171:793–799.

Submitted by: Michael Brant-Zawadzki, M.D., F.A.C.R., Hoag Memorial Hospital, Newport Beach, California; Michael Brant-Zawadzki, M.D., F.A.C.R., Senior Editor.

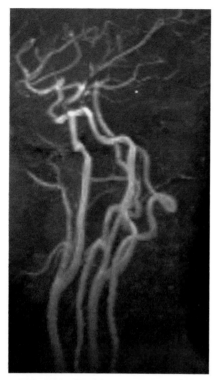

FIG. 57A. 3D TOF (FISP) 40/7/15°.

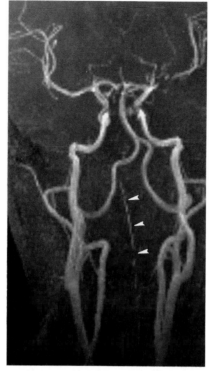

FIG. 57B. 3D TOF (FISP) 40/7/15°.

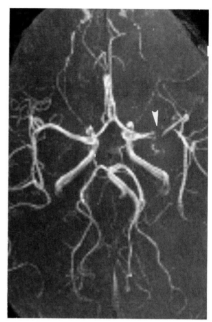

FIG. 57C. 3D TOF (FISP) 40/7/15°.

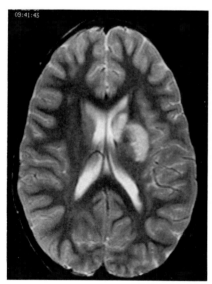

FIG. 57D. Axial SE 2800/90.

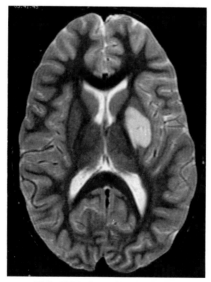

FIG. 57E. Axial SE 2800/90.

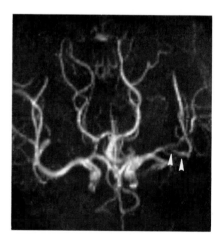

FIG. 57F. 3D TOF (FISP) 40/7/15°.

Clinical Diagnosis

A 5-year-old male, sudden onset of aphasia, and right hemiparesis with partial resolution.

Findings

The neck magnetic resonance angiography (MRA) study (Fig. 57A) reveals no abnormality of the cervical, carotid, or vertebral architecture. Normal internal carotid artery origins are shown, as well as their course to the circle of Willis. One can incidentally note a prominent central spinal artery originating off the right vertebral (Fig. 57B, *arrowheads*). However, careful attention to the intracranial circulation suggests a filling defect in the proximal middle cerebral artery on the left. The intracranial 3D time-of-flight study (Fig. 57C) verifies the presence of a "gap" (*arrowhead*) in the proximal left middle cerebral artery, as compared to the right side. The conventional spin echo T2-weighted images (Figs. 57D and E) demonstrate lesions in the caudate and lenticular nuclei, left hemisphere. Mild mass effect is seen on the adjacent ventricle.

Diagnosis

Left middle cerebral artery embolic event with infarction of the left basal ganglia.

Discussion

This child was transferred from an outlying hospital, which did not have experience with pediatric angiography. Specifically, the patient's physician wanted a noninvasive MR angiogram to help ascertain the cause of the problem. In this case, the good depiction of the cervical and intracranial vasculature provided the answer with a half-hour study time. The child went on to a full recovery. Intraarterial angiography was not done for verification; however, the clinical syndrome, the conventional MRI images, and the MR angiography study were quite convincing regarding the cause of the ischemic event. A workup for cardiac clot or septal defect proved negative. The etiology of the embolic event remains unknown.

Follow-up MRA at 3 months (Fig. 57F) shows interval partial reconstitution of the affected segment (*arrowheads*). Note that the defect in the middle cerebral artery segment is at the level of the perforating branches that would normally feed the basal ganglia. Also, note that the conventional spin-echo images demonstrate flow void in the left sylvian vessels, indicating that either collateralization or incomplete occlusion proximally had occurred. Children have relatively large perforator vessels; thus, embolic events into these branches are more common than in adults (in whom thrombotic causes of basal ganglia infarction predominate).

References

1. Rorke LB. Pathology of cerebral vascular disease in children and adolescents. In: Edward MSB, Hoffman HJ, eds. *Cerebral vascular disease in children and adolescents.* Baltimore: Williams & Wilkins, 1988;95–138.
2. Vogl TJ, Balzer JO, et al. MR angiography in children with cerebral neurovascular disease: findings in 31 cases. *AJR* 1992;159:817–823.

Submitted by: Michael Brant-Zawadzki, M.D., F.A.C.R., Hoag Memorial Hospital, Newport Beach, California; Michael Brant-Zawadzki, M.D., F.A.C.R., Senior Editor.

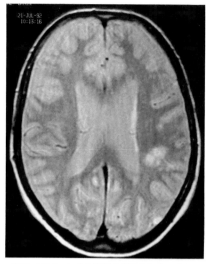

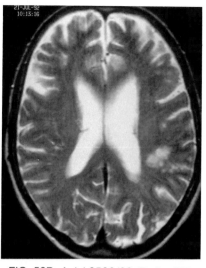

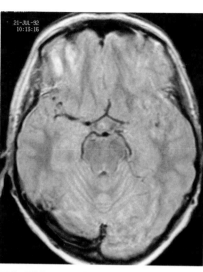

FIG. 58A. Axial 3500/19 (Turbo SE).   FIG. 58B. Axial 3500/93 (Turbo SE).   FIG. 58C. Axial SE 3500/19 (Turbo SE).

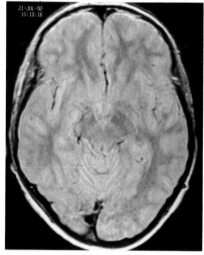

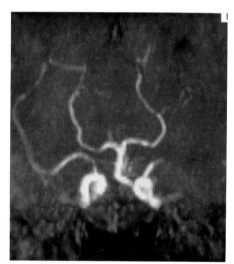

FIG. 58D. Axial SE 3500/19 (Turbo SE).   FIG. 58E. 30 TOF (FISP) 30/7/20°.

Clinical History

A 77-year-old female with left hemiparesis.

Findings

The dual echo, T2-weighted images (Figs. 58A and B) show some image degradation due to patient motion. Nevertheless, they do depict the presence of focal alteration of signal intensity in the deep left parietal region. A lower slice (Fig. 58C) shows asymmetry of the horizontal segments of the middle cerebral arteries, yet flow void in the smaller branches of the middle cerebral vessels is shown bilaterally in the operculum (Fig. 58D). MR angiogram reveals flow in the right middle cerebral artery only (Fig. 58E).

Diagnosis

Acute left middle cerebral artery occlusion with small subcortical infarction.

Discussion

The relatively small area of infarction is explained on the basis of good collateralization, which can be suspected based on the conventional spin-echo images that show good flow void in the preauricular vessels. Note that the MR angiogram does not depict these vessels as they are flowing relatively slowly, and also because a superior saturation pulse has been placed in the region of the anterior cerebrals. The anterior cerebral vessels provide the collateralization of these vessels, as shown on the intraarterial angiogram (Figs. 58F and G), which also documents the middle cerebral artery occlusion (*arrow*).

References

1. Warach S, Wei L, et al. Acute cerebral ischemia: evaluation with dynamic contrast-enhanced MR imaging and MR angiography. *Radiology* 1992;182:41–47.
2. Edelman RR, Mattle HP, et al. Magnetic resonance imaging of flow dynamics in the circle of Willis. *Stroke* 1990;21:56–65.
3. Masaryk TJ, Modic MT, et al. Intracranial circulation: preliminary clinical results with three-dimensional (volume) MR angiography. *Radiology* 1989;171:793–799.

Submitted by: Michael Brant-Zawadzki, M.D., F.A.C.R., Hoag Memorial Hospital, Newport Beach, California; Michael Brant-Zawadzki, M.D., F.A.C.R., Senior Editor.

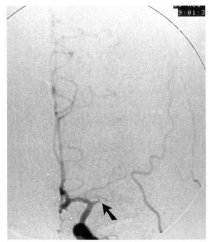

FIG. 58F. Intraarterial DSA ICA.

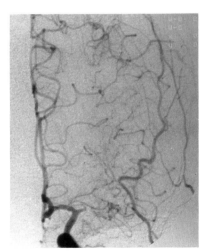

FIG. 58G. Intraarterial DSA ICA.

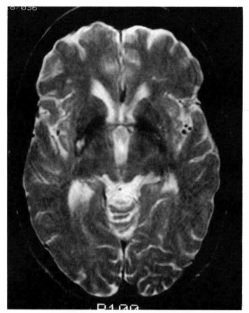

FIG. 59A. Axial SE 2800/90°.

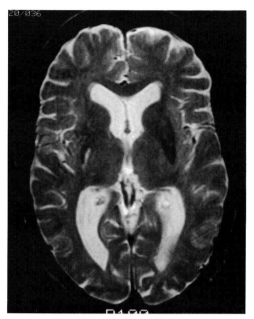

FIG. 59B. Axial SE 2800/90°.

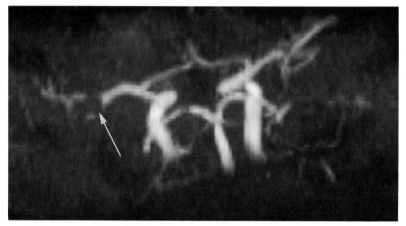

FIG. 59C. 3D TOF (FISP) 35/7/25°.

Clinical History

A 78-year-old female with sudden onset of left hemiparesis.

Findings

T2-weighted axial sections (Figs. 59A and B) demonstrate a small focus of high signal intensity in the right lenticular nucleus, bordering the posterior limb of the internal capsule. No other abnormalities were detected on this study. The MR angiogram (Fig. 59C) demonstrates a region of flow void (*arrow*) in the region of the right middle cerebral artery trifurcation, with diminished flow distally.

Diagnosis

Basal ganglia infarct due to saddle embolus in the right middle cerebral artery.

Discussion

This early generation MR angiogram demonstrates its value in identifying the etiology of a stroke. This patient had normal carotid artery bifurcations documented by both MRA and intraarterial angiography. The intraarterial angiogram verifies the filling defect (*arrow*) in the right middle cerebral artery (Fig. 59D). The patient was on estrogen replacement therapy, and the likely cause of the embolus was a hypercoagulable state. The MR angiogram exaggerates the degree of vessel occlusion secondary to dephasing of turbulent flow spins.

References

1. Warach S, Li W, et al. Acute cerebral ischemia: evaluation with dynamic contrast-enhanced MR imaging and MR angiography. *Radiology* 1992;182:41–47.
2. Masaryk TJ, Modic MT, et al. Intracranial circulation: preliminary clinical results with three-dimensional (volume) MR angiography. *Radiology* 1989;171:793–799.

Submitted by: Michael Brant-Zawadzki, M.D., F.A.C.R., Hoag Memorial Hospital, Newport Beach, California; Michael Brant-Zawadzki, M.D., F.A.C.R., Senior Editor.

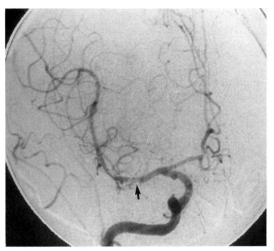

FIG. 59D. Intraarterial angiogram DSA RCA.

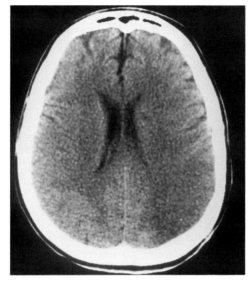

FIG. 60A. Axial CT.

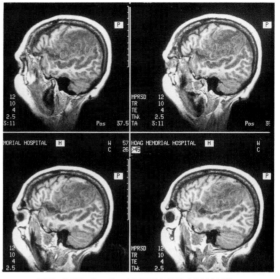

FIG. 60B. Sagittal MPRAGE 10/4/12°.

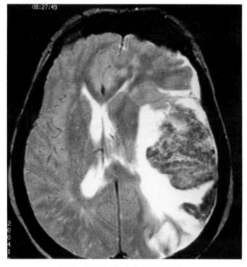

FIG. 60C. Axial 2500/90.

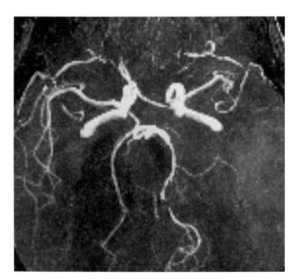

FIG. 60D. 3D TOF (FISP) 40/7/15°.

Clinical History

A 59-year-old female with acute right hemiparesis and aphasia.

Findings

CT scan (Fig. 60A) obtained on day of admission shows a large, wedge-shaped area of low density in the posterior left middle cerebral artery distribution. T1-weighted sagittal images (Fig. 60B), as well as the T2-weighted axial image (Fig. 60C) obtained 2 days later show hemorrhagic conversion of the large bland infarct. Note the increasing mass effect on this study. The MR angiogram (Fig. 60D) demonstrates loss of flow in the distal branches of the left middle cerebral artery. Note the medial deviation of the posterior cerebral artery in the ambient cistern, indicating transtentorial herniation from the mass effect.

Diagnosis

Left middle cerebral artery embolic infarct with hemorrhagic conversion and resulting transtentorial herniation.

Discussion

This case demonstrates the typical evolution of a large embolic infarction in the left middle cerebral artery distribution. The initial infarct shows relatively little mass effect due to loss of perfusion. With reflow following clot lysis, the resulting damage of the microvascular bed allows massive vasogenic edema and breakthrough bleeding. This may produce evolution of the infarct to the degree shown here, worsening of the patient's clinical status, and potentially lethal consequences on the basis of herniation.

References

1. Warach S, Wei L, et al. Acute cerebral ischemia: evaluation with dynamic contrast enhanced MR imaging and MR angiography. *Radiology* 1992;182:41–47.
2. Heiserman JE, Drayer BP, et al. Intracranial vascular stenosis and occlusion: evaluation with three-dimensional time-of-flight MR angiography. *Radiology* 1992;185:667–673.
3. Brant-Zawadzki M, Pereira B, et al. MR imaging of acute experimental ischemia in cats. *AJNR* 1986;7:7–11.

Submitted by: Michael Brant-Zawadzki, M.D., F.A.C.R., Hoag Memorial Hospital, Newport Beach, California; Michael Brant-Zawadzki, M.D., F.A.C.R., Senior Editor.

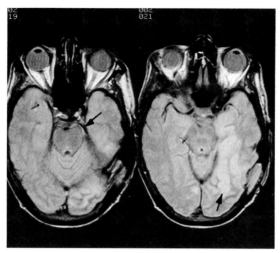

FIG. 61A. SE 2100/30.

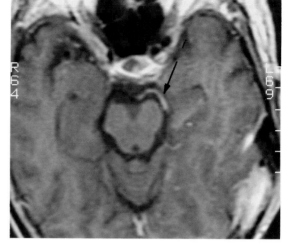

FIG. 61B. SE 500/20.

Clinical History

A 59-year-old male with lung primary presents with homonymous hemianopia.

Findings

Axial proton density images demonstrate hyperintense signal in the left temporoparietal occipital lobe, left proximal posterior cerebral artery (PCA), and left temporoparietal epidural space and calvarium. (Fig. 61A, *arrows*). Gadolinium [(Gd)-DTPA] contrast-enhanced T1-weighted image shows intravascular enhancement of the left PCA (Fig. 61B, *arrow*) and the left calvarial/epidural lesions (Fig. 61B). The occipital lobe parenchymal signal is without contrast enhancement.

Diagnosis

Acute left PCA infarct and left calvarial metastasis with epidural extension.

Discussion

Recent reports have documented that one of the earliest signs of acute cerebral infarction is intravascular enhancement from presumed slow arterial flow and the loss of time-of-flight arterial signal void (1–3). Arterial flow kinetics may be influenced by maximal vasodilation, arteriolar-capillary block, and diminished regional flow (1). Arterial enhancement with Gd-DTPA can preceed parenchymal T2 signal abnormality as well as parenchymal enhancement due to blood-brain barrier breakdown and tends not to be visualized beyond the eighth day after infarction. Larger infarcts can also be accompanied after 1 to 3 days by meningeal or dural enhancement (1). In this case tumor metastasis accounts for the dural enhancement.

References

1. Elster AD, Moody DM. Early cerebral infarction: gadopentetate dimeglumine enhancement. *Radiology* 1990;177:627–632.
2. Sato A, Takahashi S, Soma Y, et al. Cerebral infarction: early detection by means of contrast-enhanced cerebral arteries at MR imaging. *Radiology* 1991;178:433–439.
3. Crain MR, Yuh WTC, Greene GM, et al. Cerebral ischemia: evaluation with contrast-enhanced MR imaging. *AJNR* 1991;12:631–639.

Submitted by: Orest B. Boyko, M.D., Ph.D., Duke University Medical Center, Durham, North Carolina; Michael Brant-Zawadzki, M.D., F.A.C.R., Senior Editor.

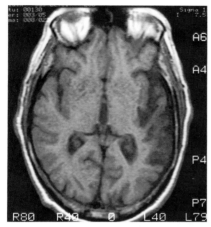

FIG. 62A. SE 500/20.

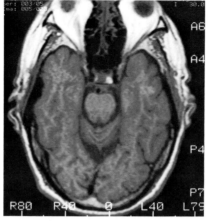

FIG. 62B. SE 500/20.

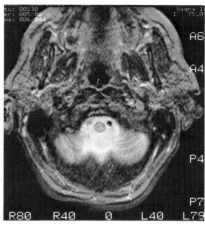

FIG. 62C. SE 2300/80.

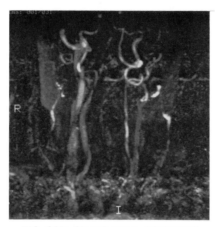

FIG. 62D. 2D PC MRA, 32/10/45°.

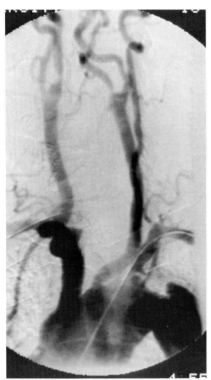

FIG. 62E. Conventional arch angiogram.

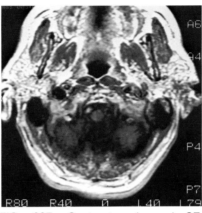

FIG. 62F. Contrast enhanced SE 500/20.

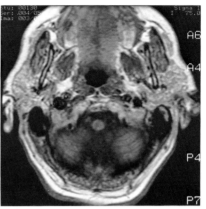

FIG. 62G. Contrast enhanced SE 500/20.

Clinical History

A 72-year-old male with past history of stroke.

Findings

An old left middle cerebral artery (MCA) stroke (Fig. 62A) is present with normal caliber and flow void of the left internal carotid artery (ICA) (Fig. 62B) on T1-weighted images. There is no flow void in the right vertebral artery (VA) on T2-weighted image (Fig. 62C). No signal abnormality is present in the brain stem. The 2D phase contrast (PC) magnetic resonance angiography (MRA) shows absent flow in the right vertebral artery (Fig. 62D) (velocity encoding of 45 cm/sec). Conventional digital arch angiogram (Fig. 62C) shows occlusion of the right vertebral artery at its origin. Curiously, on the contrast-enhanced T1-weighted image the occluded right VA shows homogeneous enhancement when compared with the precontrast image (Figs. 62F and G).

Diagnosis

Old left MCA stroke with asymptomatic occlusion of the right vertebral artery at its origin.

Discussion

The MR signal intensities of intravascular thrombus differ from those of extravascular hematoma or venous thrombus (1). Arterial thrombus, as illustrated by this case in the right VA, has signal intensity isointense to brain on T1-, proton-density, and T2-weighted images (1) with complete loss of normal flow void (1,2). These signal characteristics of arterial thrombi are reflected in their histopathology of containing mainly fibrin and platelets and lacking the hemoglobin-containing red blood cells (RBCs), which contribute to higher signal intensity (1). Venous thrombus or extravascular hematoma contains a large amount of RBCs and takes on MR signal characteristics reflective of the oxidation state of hemoglobin (hyperintense signal relative to brain due to methemoglobin).

The enhancement of arteries on T1-weighted images has been described as an early sign of infarction or ischemia and is thought to represent a slowing of arterial circulation (3). As this case illustrates, an occluded artery and the associated thrombus can enhance. Contrast may get into an occluded vessel via recanalized portions of the clot, percolation of contrast through the vasa vasorum into the clot, retrograde flow, or anastomtic collaterals (4).

148

References

1. Katz BH, Quencer RM, Kaplan JO, et al. MR imaging of intracranial carotid occlusion. *AJNR* 1989;10:345–350.
2. Brant-Zawadzki M. Routine MR imaging of the internal carotid artery siphon: angiographic correlation with cervical carotid lesions. *AJNR* 1990;11:467–471.
3. Elster AD, Moody DM. Early cerebral infarction: gadopentetate dimeglumine enhancement. *Radiology* 1990;177:627–632.
4. Boyko OB. Gadolinium-DTPA enhancement of intraarterial thrombus. Book of Abstracts, American Society of Neuroradiology, 28th Annual Meeting, March 1990.

Submitted by: Orest B. Boyko, M.D., Ph.D., Duke University Medical Center, Durham, North Carolina; Michael Brant-Zawadzki, M.D., F.A.C.R., Senior Editor.

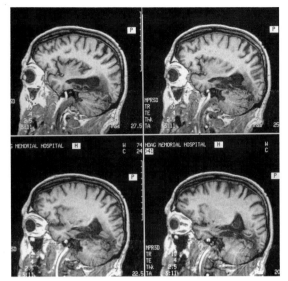

FIG. 63A. Sagittal 3D (MPRAGE) 10/4/12°.

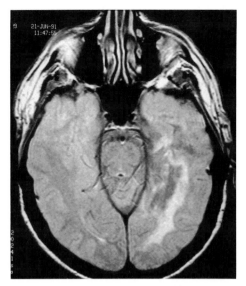

FIG. 63B. Axial 2500/22.

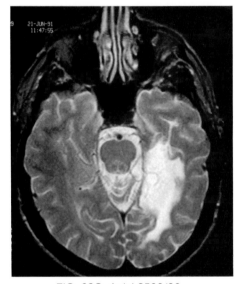

FIG. 63C. Axial 2500/90.

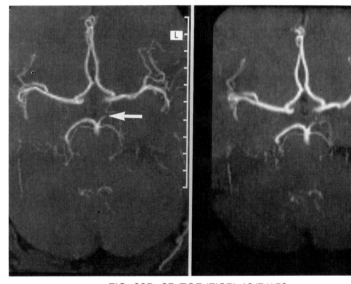

FIG. 63D. 3D TOF (FISP) 40/7/15°.

Clinical History

A 61-year-old male with right quadrant hemianopia.

Findings

The contiguous thin-section T1-weighted sagittal images (MP RAGE) (Fig. 63A) show diffuse low signal intensity in the inframedial region of the left temporal lobe extending to the occipital lobe. The T2-weighted axial sequence (Figs. 63B and C) depict the high signal alteration of the brain in the same location. The 3D time-of-flight magnetic resonance angiogram (MRA) (Fig. 63D) shows attenuation of the left posterior cerebral artery (*arrow*). The cervical portion of the MR angiogram (Fig. 63E) depicts absence of the right vertebral artery.

Diagnosis

Left mesiotemporal and occipital infarction, most likely on the basis of vertebral occlusive disease and subsequent embolization.

Discussion

The value of conventional MRI in conjunction with MRA is shown here. The end-organ damage depicted with routine spin echo MR imaging can be explained on a vascular basis as elucidated by the MR angiographic portion of the study. Although the cause of right vertebral occlusion cannot be discerned on this study, the visualization of the cervicocranial vessels aids in patient management as no further workup need be done. If, on the other hand, a small vertebral or irregular basilar were shown, an intraarterial angiogram may have been performed to evaluate for possible embolic source along the blood flow pathway into the posterior circulation.

References

1. Warach S, Li W, et al. Acute cerebral ischemia: evaluation with dynamic contrast-enhanced MR imaging and MR angiography. *Radiology* 1992;182:41–47.
2. Masaryk TJ, Modic MT, et al. Intracranial circulation: preliminary clinical results with three dimensional (volume) MR angiography. *Radiology* 1989;171:793–799.

Submitted by: Michael Brant-Zawadzki, M.D., F.A.C.R., Hoag Memorial Hospital, Newport Beach, California; Michael Brant-Zawadzki, M.D., F.A.C.R., Senior Editor.

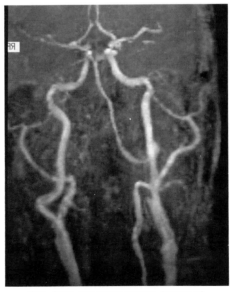

FIG. 63E. 2D TOF (FISP) 40/7/15°.

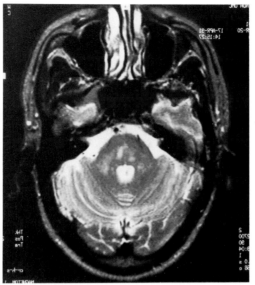

FIG. 64A. Axial SE 2700/90.

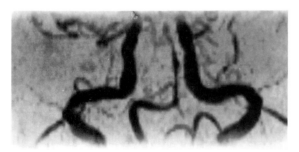

FIG. 64B. 3D TOF FISP TR = 40, TE = 7, FA = 25°.

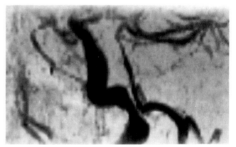

FIG. 64C. 3D TOF FISP TR = 40, TE = 7, FA = 25°.

Clinical History

A 71-year-old with pontine ischemia symptoms.

Findings

T2-weighted image (Fig. 64A) at the level of the pons demonstrates several abnormal small foci of high signal intensity. The 3D time-of-flight angiogram demonstrates diffuse basilar irregularity and narrowing on both the frontal and lateral projections (Figs. 64B and C, respectively).

Diagnosis

Atherosclerotic basilar disease with resulting pontine infarction.

Discussion

The vertebral basilar intraarterial angiography is relatively more hazardous than carotid intraarterial angiography; thus, the ability to noninvasively evaluate the vertebral basilar system in patients with brain stem symptoms is a clear virtue of MR angiography (MRA). Note that the etiology of the disease process here cannot be fully evaluated, although given the age of the patient and the clinical setting, it is likely to be atherosclerotic rather than on the basis of other causes (such as spasm, vasculitis, etc.). It appears that the left vertebral artery is either occluded or has very slow flow, given its poor visualization on the MRA studies.

References

1. Wagle WA, Dumoulin CL, et al. 3DFT MR angiography of carotid and basilar arteries. *AJNR* 1989;10:911–919.
2. Warach S, Li W, et al. Acute cerebral ischemia: evaluation with dynamic contrast-enhanced MR imaging and MR angiography. *Radiology* 1992;182:41–47.
3. Masaryk TJ, Modic MT, et al. Intracranial circulation: preliminary clinical results with three dimensional (volume) MR angiography. *Radiology* 1989;171:793–799.

Submitted by: Anton N. Hasso, M.D., F.A.C.R., Loma Linda University School of Medicine, Loma Linda, California; Michael Brant-Zawadzki, M.D., F.A.C.R., Senior Editor.

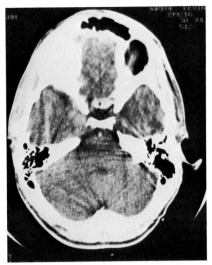

FIG. 65A. Noncontrast CT scan.

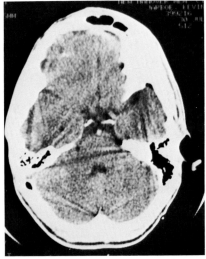

FIG. 65B. Noncontrast CT scan.

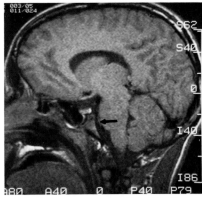

FIG. 65C. Sagittal SE 500/20.

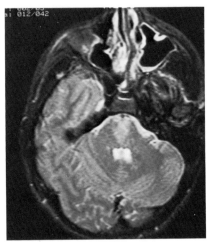

FIG. 65D. SE 3200/80.

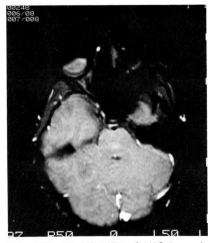

FIG. 65E. 2D PC MRA, 24/13 (magnitude image).

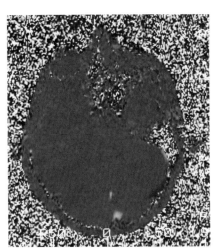

FIG. 65F. 2D PC MRA, 24/13 (phase image).

Clinical History

A 15-year-old male with loss of consciousness 8 hours after being hit in the head with a surfboard.

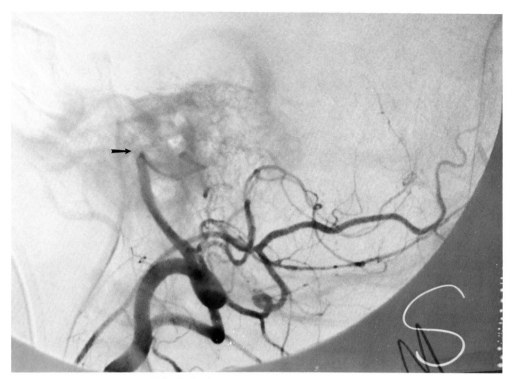

FIG. 65G. Conventional left VA angiogram.

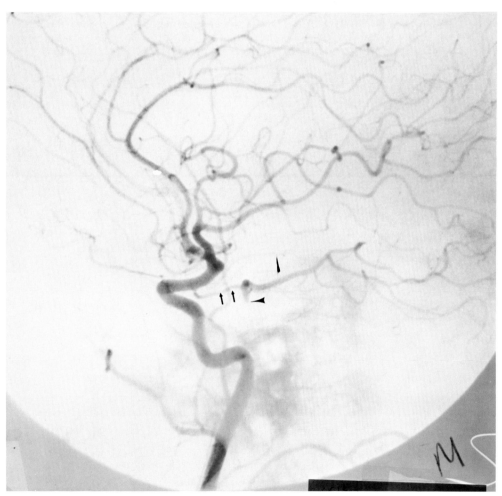

FIG. 65H. Conventional left CCA angiogram.

Findings

Noncontrast CT scan (Fig. 65A) shows dense basilar artery (BA) with streak artifact over the pons, but the BA tip has normal attenuation (Fig. 65B). The dense basilar artery shows signal isointense with brain and lack of a flow void (Fig. 65C, *arrow*). T2-weighted image 1 day later shows hypointense signal in the same segment of the basilar artery suggesting flow void or deoxyhemoglobin in a thrombus mimicking flow (Fig. 65D) with hyperintense signal or ischemia or infarction in the pons. The 2D phase contrast (PC) magnetic resonance angiography (MRA) shows lack of flow-related enhancement (FRE) in the basilar artery on the magnitude image (Fig. 65E), confirmed on the phase image (Fig. 65F) using a velocity encoding of 80 cm/sec.

Conventional left vertebral artery (VA) angiogram shows occlusion of the BA at the level of the anterior inferior cerebellar artery (Fig. 65G, *arrow*). Left common carotid artery (CCA) conventional angiogram shows the patent left posterior communicating artery (Fig. 65H, *arrows*) with a patent BA tip and reflux of contrast into the distal BA to the level of the occlusion (Fig. 65H, *arrowhead*).

Diagnosis

Spontaneous occlusion and thrombosis of the basilar artery with pontine infarct.

Discussion

Incidental head trauma may have contributed to the BA thrombosis, but an actual point of dissection cannot be identified. Atherosclerosis is most often associated with BA occlusion (1,3). The earliest abnormality is the absence of flow void on T2-weighted images, seen sometimes within 90 minutes (1). This case illustrates that at 24 to 48 hours deoxyhemoglobin thrombus causes decreased signal intensity and can mimic flow void on T2-weighted images. Both T1-weighted and 2D PC MRA can be used to suggest the presence of thrombus (2).

References

1. Knepper L, Biller J, Adams HP, et al. MR imaging of basilar artery occlusion. *J Comput Assist Tomogr* 1990;14:32–35.
2. Nadel L, Braun IF, Kraft, et al. Intracranial vascular abnormalities: value of MR phase imaging to distinguish thrombus from flowing blood. *AJNR* 1991;11:1133–1140.
3. Kubik CS, Adams RD. Occlusion of basilar artery—clinical and pathological study. *Brain* 1946;69:6–121.

Submitted by: Orest B. Boyko, M.D., Ph.D., Duke University Medical Center, Durham, North Carolina; Michael Brant-Zawadzki, M.D., F.A.C.R., Senior Editor.

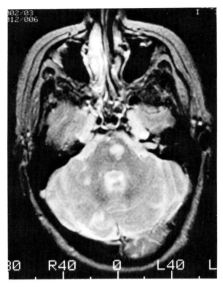

FIG. 66A. SE 2100/80.

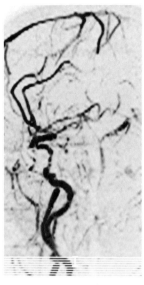

FIG. 66B. 2D TOF MRA (GRE 45/9/60°) 3-D reprojection lateral.

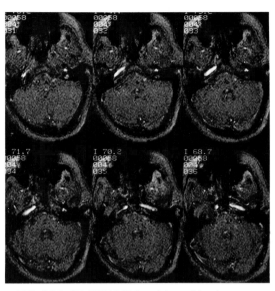

FIG. 66C. 2D TOF MRA axial partition images.

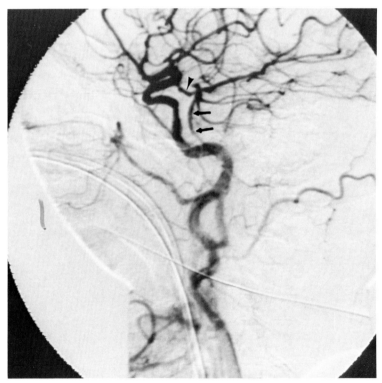

FIG. 66D. Lateral conventional RCCA angiogram.

Clinical History

A 61-year-old female with left facial numbness and cerebellar ataxia.

Findings

Axial T2-weighted image shows abnormal signal intensity in the pons and cerebellum secondary to ischemic change (Fig. 66A). The basilar artery has diminished caliber (Fig. 66A). Lateral projection 2D time-of-flight (TOF) magnetic resonance angiography (MRA) demonstrates poor visualization of the basilar artery (only the distal signal is seen at all). Individual partition images show decreased caliber of the BA with minimal bright signal intensity indicating decreased FRE in the BA (Fig. 66C). Conventional right common carotid angiogram (CCA) shows retrograde filling of the distal BA (Fig. 66D, *arrows*) through a patent posterior communicating artery (Fig. 66D, *arrowhead*).

Diagnosis

Vertebralbasilar insufficiency (VBI) with infarction due to atherosclerosis.

Discussion

Clinical findings of VBI are broad including vertigo, ataxia, deafness, nystagmus, ophthalmoplegia, bilateral body dysesthesias or corticospinal-tract signs. In MRA the individual partition images that are used to make the 3D reprojections should always be reviewed for flow in a vessel when using the maximum intensity pixel (MIP) algorithm. Signal dropout of FRE in a vessel in the MIP 3D reprojection images has been reported (2) and is demonstrated by this case. In addition a routine superiorly placed saturation pulse was used to negate venous flow. However, because of the retrograde flow in the BA, flow in this artery is also superior/inferior (in the direction of venous outflow) and would be susceptible to the saturation pulse and cause loss of FRE (particularly if the saturation pulse "travels" with the individual slice acquisition).

References

1. Williams D, Wilson TG. The diagnosis of the major and minor syndromes of basilar insufficiency. *Brain* 1952;85:741–774.
2. Anderson CM, Saloner D, Tsuruda JS, et al. Artifacts in maximum-intensity-projection display MR angiograms. *AJR* 1990;154:623–629.

Submitted by: Orest B. Boyko, M.D., Ph.D., Duke University Medical Center, Durham, North Carolina; Michael Brant-Zawadzki, M.D., F.A.C.R., Senior Editor.

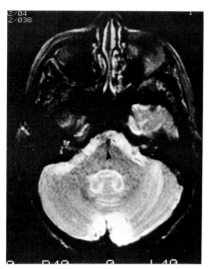

FIG. 67A. SE 2000/80.

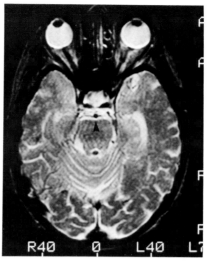

FIG. 67B. SE 2000/80.

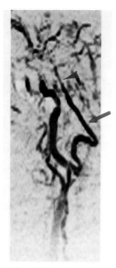

FIG. 67C. 2D TOF MRA (45/9/60°) lateral 3D reprojection.

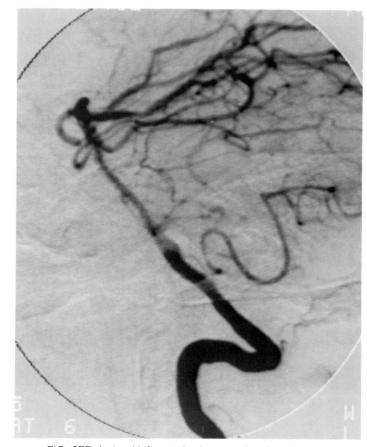

FIG. 67D. Lateral left vertebral conventional angiogram.

Clinical History

An 81-year-old female presents with dysarthria, vertigo, nausea, and vomiting.

Findings

T2-weighted image demonstrates no signal abnormality in the pons or cerebellar white matter (Fig. 67A). Basilar artery (BA) flow void is present (Fig. 67A, *arrowhead*). More distal image demonstrates decreased caliber of the BA (Fig. 67B, *arrowhead*) without any associated brain stem signal abnormality.

The 2D time-of-flight (TOF) magnetic resonance angiography (MRA) 3D reprojection shows in the lateral projection normal caliber of the proximal BA (Fig. 67C, *arrow*) and decreasing circumferential caliber of the distal BA (Fig. 67C, *arrowhead*). Conventional vertebral artery angiography confirms the MRA findings (Fig. 67D).

Diagnosis

Vertebral basilar insufficiency (VBI) due to atherosclerosis of the BA.

Discussion

VBI is a common cause of vertigo but it is unclear whether the cause is due to ischemia of the labyrinth or of the brain stem. As this case illustrates there can be abnormal vessel caliber with normal flow void present with no associated parenchymal signal abnormality in the posterior fossa. The 2D TOF MRA adequately demonstrated the tapered appearance of the middle and upper third of the basilar artery due to atherosclerosis, which was suggested by the caliber change on the T2-weighted images.

References

1. Williams D, Wilson TG. The diagnosis of the major and minor syndromes of basilar insufficiency. *Brain* 1962;85:741–774.
2. Keller PJ, Drayer BF, Fram EK, et al. MR angiography with two-dimensional acquisition and three-dimensional display—works in progress. *Radiology* 1989;173:527–532.

Submitted by: Orest B. Boyko, M.D., Ph.D., Duke University Medical Center, Durham, North Carolina; Michael Brant-Zawadzki, M.D., F.A.C.R., Senior Editor.

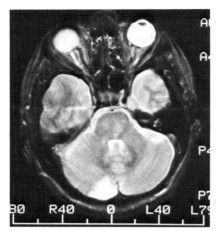

FIG. 68A. SE 2800/80.

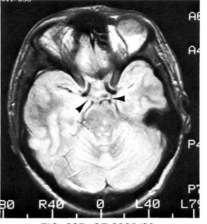

FIG. 68B. SE 2800/30.

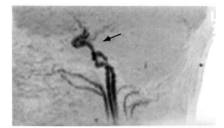

FIG. 68C. 3D TOF MRA (60/7/20°) 3D reprojection.

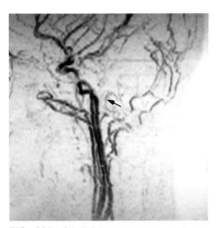

FIG. 68D. 2D TOF MRA (50/9/60°) 3D reprojection.

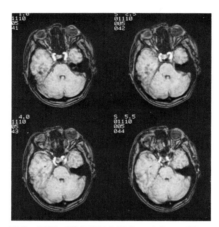

FIG. 68E. 3D TOF MRA axial partition images.

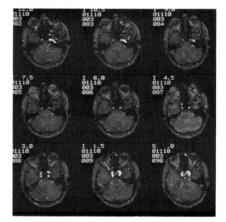

FIG. 68F. 2D TOF MRA axial partition images.

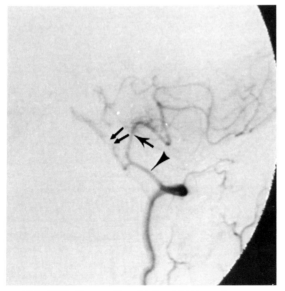

FIG. 68G. Conventional lateral LVA angiogram.

Clinical History

A 36-year-old female presents clinically with locked-in syndrome.

Findings

Axial T2-weighted image (Fig. 68A) shows two confluent areas of hyperintense signal in the pons and a right cerebellar hemisphere lesion. The basilar artery (BA) has flow void but decreased caliber. Note hyperintense signal in the left midbrain on proton density image but well-developed bilateral posterior communicating arteries (Fig. 68B, *arrowheads*). The 3D time-of-flight (TOF) magnetic resonance angiography (MRA) demonstrates no flow-related enhancement (FRE) in the BA (Fig. 68C, *arrow*). The BA is not identified on 2D TOF MRA but the left posterior inferior cerebellar artery (PICA) can be seen (Fig. 68D, *arrow*). The axial input slices demonstrate poor FRE of the BA on 3D TOF MRA (Fig. 68E) and 2D TOF MRA (Fig. 68F) with decreased vessel caliber. Conventional angiogram of the left vertebral artery (VA) shows in a lateral projection a narrowed VA (Fig. 68G, *arrowhead*) normal PICA (Fig. 68G, *arrow*) and abnormally narrowed BA (Fig. 68G, *double arrow*).

Diagnosis

Vertebral basilar insufficiency (VBI) from BA occlusive disease of unknown cause.

Discussion

Locked-in syndrome results from pontine infarction usually of the pontine base with sparing of vertical eye movements. Patients are tetraparetic and mute but do comprehend their environment (1).

Regular spin-echo images demonstrate infarction as areas of hyperintense signal and the decreased BA flow as a diminished vessel caliber. Due to slow flow and saturation effects (2), the BA may not be identified on the 3D MRA reprojections simulating complete occlusion, although some FRE can be identified on individual partition images. The presence of flow void on SE images confirms BA patency.

References

1. Kemper TL, Romanul FCA. State resembling akinetic mutism in basilar artery thrombosis. *Neurology* 1967;17:74.
2. Turski P, Bernstein M, Boyko OB, et al. *Vascular magnetic resonance imaging.* GE Medical Systems Application Guide, Milwaukee, WI, 1990.

Submitted by: Orest B. Boyko, M.D., Ph.D., Duke University Medical Center, Durham, North Carolina; Michael Brant-Zawadzki, M.D., F.A.C.R., Senior Editor.

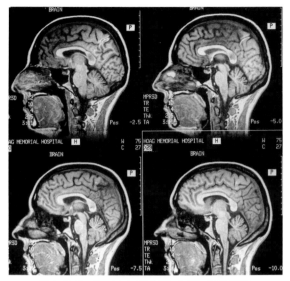

FIG. 69A. Sagittal 3D MPRAGE 10/4/12°.

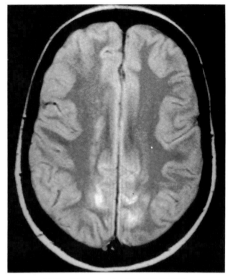

FIG. 69B. Axial SE 2500/22.

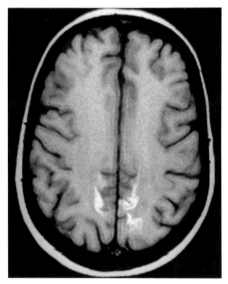

FIG. 69C. Axial SE 720/22.

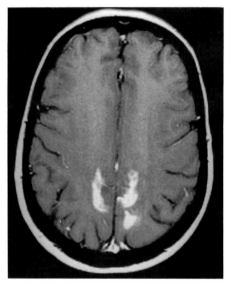

FIG. 69D. Postcontrast axial SE 720/22.

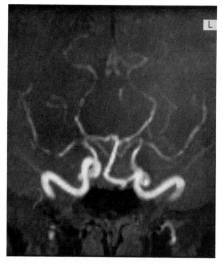

FIG. 69E. 3D TOF (FISP) 30/7/20°.

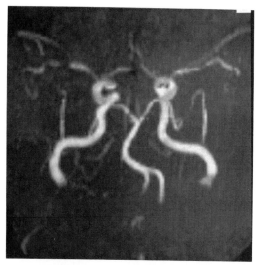

FIG. 69F. 3D TOF (FISP) 30/7/20°.

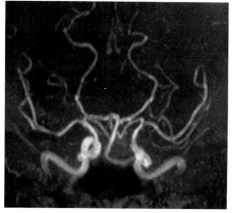

FIG. 69G. 3D TOF 42/7/20° MTS/TONE.

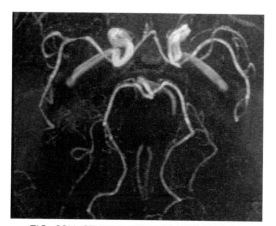

FIG. 69H. 3D TOF 42/7/20° MTS/TONE.

Clinical History

A 46-year-old female with history of inflammatory bowel disease, now presents with transient right and left hemiparesis and headaches.

Findings

MR images demonstrate a focal lesion in the splenium of the corpus callosum (Fig. 69A). Axial first echo image (Fig. 69B) demonstrates bilateral white matter abnormalities close to the gray-white matter junction. The pre- and postcontrast T1-weighted images (Figs. 69C and D) demonstrate that these are hemorrhagic foci that do exhibit some enhancement.

An MR angiogram (MRA) was performed, which demonstrates multifocal areas of stenosis in the major intracranial vessels, particularly in the posterior and middle cerebral artery distribution (Figs. 69E and F).

Diagnosis

Intracranial large vessel vasculitis.

Discussion

Multifocal lesions are the hallmark of vasculitis, particularly in a gray-white junction distribution with a hemorrhagic component. The differential diagnosis of vasculitis includes infectious and noninfectious inflammatory conditions, as well as neoplastic causes such as leptomeningeal tumor. With new techniques, small vessel delineation in the brain on MRA has improved. In this particular case, the follow-up study was done with high-resolution (512) matrix, a variable flip angle, as well as background suppression through use of magnetization transfer suppression pulses (Figs. 69G and H). The lesions responded over time to steroid therapy. The association between systemic vasculitis (including cerebral) and inflammatory bowel disease is a well-recognized yet poorly understood phenomenon. Since this patient has no other underlying etiology for vasculitis, it was thought to be possibly related in this case.

References

1. Edelman RR, Ahn SS, et al. Improved time-of-flight MR angiography with magnetization transfer contrast. *Radiology* 1992;184:395–399.
2. Nelson J, Barron MM, et al. Cerebral vasculitis and ulcerative colitis. *Neurology* 1986;36:719–721.
3. Lee JT. Vasculitis and the gut: unwilling partners or strange bedfellows. *J Rheumatol* 1991;18(5):647–648.
4. Danzi JT. Extraintestinal manifestations of idiopathic inflammatory bowel disease. *Arch Intern Med* 1988;148:297–301.

Submitted by: Michael Brant-Zawadzki, M.D., F.A.C.R., Hoag Memorial Hospital, Newport Beach, California; Michael Brant-Zawadzki, M.D., F.A.C.R., Senior Editor.

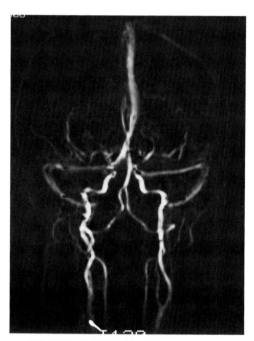

FIG. 70A. 2D PC MRA (25/12, TR/TE).

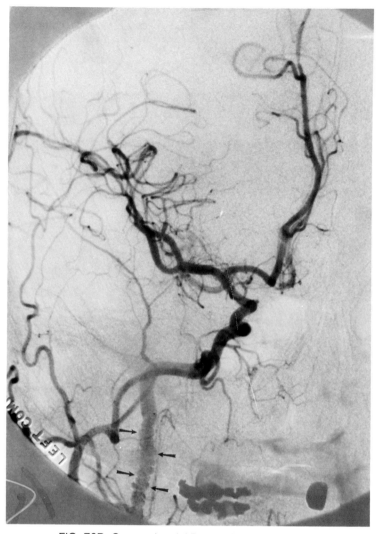

FIG. 70B. Conventional AP right CCA angiogram.

Clinical History

A 42-year-old female with transient left hemiparesis.

Findings

The 2D phase contrast (PC) magnetic resonance angiography (MRA) (1) demonstrates bilateral corrugated cervical internal carotid arteries (ICAs) (Fig. 70A, *arrows*). Conventional right common carotid angiogram (Fig. 70B, *arrows*) confirms the string-of-beads appearance.

Diagnosis

Bilateral fibromuscular dysplasia (FMD).

Discussion

FMD usually involves the renal arteries and, when affecting the ICA, is usually bilateral (2). There is an increased incidence of intracranial aneurysm. The corrugated appearance of the ICA must be distinguished from stationary arterial waves that are more regularly spaced than those of FMD with less luminal narrowing.

References

1. Dumoulin CL, Hart HR. MR angiography. *Radiology* 1986;61:717–720.
2. Houser OW, Baker HL. Fibromuscular dysplasia and other uncommon diseases of the cervical carotid artery: angiographic aspects. *Am J Roentgenol Radium Ther Nucl Med* 1968;104:201–212.

Submitted by: Orest B. Boyko, M.D., Ph.D., Duke University Medical Center, Durham, North Carolina; Michael Brant-Zawadzki, M.D., F.A.C.R., Senior Editor.

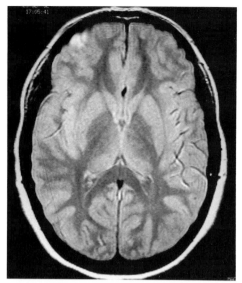

FIG. 71A. Axial SE 2500/22.

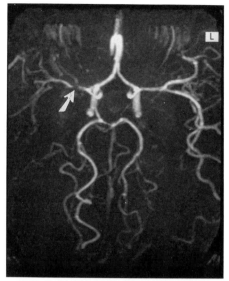

FIG. 71B. 3D TOF (FISP) 40/7/15°.

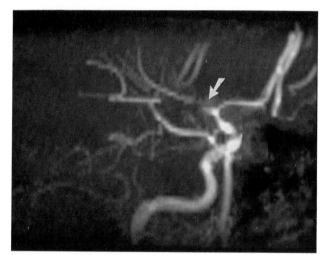

FIG. 71C. 3D TOF (FISP) 40/7/15°.

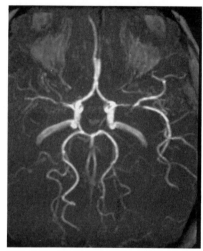

FIG. 71D. 3D TOF (FISP) 40/7/15° obtained 2 weeks later.

Clinical History

A 25-year-old female with history of migraine, now presents with unusually painful right-sided headache without neurological deficit.

Findings

Conventional MR image at the level of the third ventricle shows no abnormality (Fig. 71A). (High signal in the right frontal lobe represents partial volume artifact from the orbital fat.) In fact, the entire brain MRI study was normal. Magnetic resonance angiography (MRA) demonstrates clear asymmetry of the right middle cerebral artery complex when compared with the left (Fig. 71B). In retrospect, this is also seen on the conventional MR image. There is a focal stenosis in what appears to be the proximal middle cerebral artery segment (Fig. 71B, *arrow*). Oblique view (Fig. 71C, *arrow*) demonstrates this to further advantage. Because the finding was unusual, a repeat study was done 2 weeks later (Fig. 71D), when the migraine resolved, showing no interval change.

Diagnosis

Presumed focal dissection of middle cerebral artery.

Discussion

Focal intracranial large vessel dissections are quite uncommon. They can occur in the setting of trauma or intense physical exertion (no such history was obtained in this patient). They may also be predisposed to by high blood pressure, atherosclerotic disease, as well as congenital weakness of the vessel. Migraine headaches have a reported association with cerebral arterial dissections. Intraarterial angiogram (Figs. 71E and F) verifies the lesion. The treatment course in this patient included chronic anticoagulation. Again, no focal neurologic symptom was encountered during her course of management.

Acquired lesions such as vasculitis would be expected to produce multifocal abnormalities. Congenital lesions, such as localized moyamoya, would be expected to develop a prominent collateralization pattern by this time. The spasm, perhaps related to migraine, is generally not known to effect large vessels such as this, particularly in a focal fashion; however, that possibility was considered but ruled out by the follow-up study.

References

1. Hart RG, Easton JD. Dissections of cervical and cerebral arteries. *Neurol Clin* 1983;1(1):155–182.
2. Linden MD, Chou SM, et al. Cerebral arterial dissection. *Cleve Clin J Med* 1987;54:105–114.
3. Heiserman JE, Drayer BP, et al. Intracranial vascular stenosis and occlusion: evaluation of three-dimensional time-of-flight MR angiography. *Radiology* 1992;185:667–673.

Submitted by: Michael Brant-Zawadzki, M.D., F.A.C.R., Hoag Memorial Hospital, Newport Beach, California; Michael Brant-Zawadzki, M.D., F.A.C.R., Senior Editor.

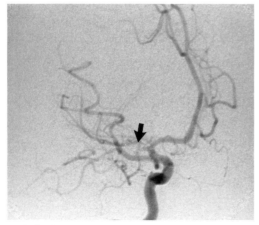

FIG. 71E. Intraarterial DSA RCA injection.

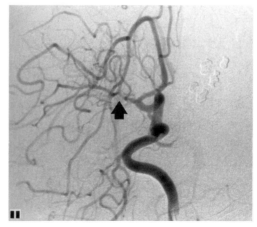

FIG. 71F. Intraarterial DSA RCA injection.

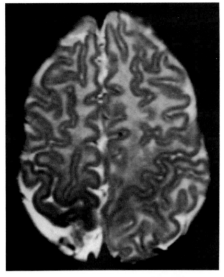

FIG. 72A. Axial SE 3500/90.

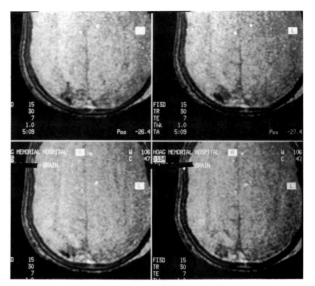

FIG. 72B. 3D TOF (FISP) 30/7/15°.

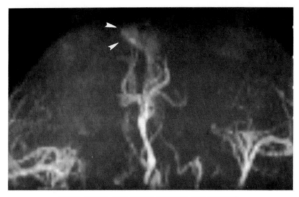

FIG. 72C. 3D TOF (FISP) 30/7/15°.

Clinical History

A 5-month-old infant with seizures and port-wine nevus on face.

Findings

The MRI study on this infant demonstrates focal atrophy in the right parietal region on the T2-weighted image (Fig. 72A). Selected partitions utilizing the gradient recalled FISP 3D technique (the basis for the MR angiographic views) shows focal area of signal loss in the same region (Fig. 72B). The maximum intensity projections of the partitions at higher level to the atrophy shows a blushing lesion over the convexity, just to the right of midline (Fig. 72C).

Diagnosis

Sturge-Weber syndrome (also known as encephalotrigeminal angiomatosis).

Discussion

The constellation of findings are classic for this type of congenital neurocutaneous syndrome. Children with Sturge-Weber syndrome have angiomatous malformations affecting the face, choroid of the eye, and leptomeninges. Cortical calcification is characteristic and is best demonstrated by CT scanning—although it can also be easily seen with MR, particularly when gradient echo sequences are utilized. The pial angiomatosis does exhibit high perfusion, and thus is easily depicted with MR angiographic technique. Presumably the combination of vascular steal phenomenon and chronic seizures contribute to the atrophy in the involved region of the brain, and, in time, result in hemihypertrophy of the ipsilateral cavarium, paranasal sinuses, and mastoid air cells.

References

1. Wasenko JJ, Rosenblum SA, et al. The Sturge-Weber syndrome: comparison of MR and CT characteristics. *AJNR* 1990;11:131–134.
2. Barkovich AJ. Phakomatoses. In: Barkovich AJ, ed. *Contemporary neuroimaging: Vol 1. Pediatric neuroimaging.* New York: Raven Press, 1990;123–147.
3. Byrd SE. Central nervous system manifestation of inherited disorders. In: Atlas SW, ed. *Magnetic resonance imaging of the brain and spine.* New York: Raven Press, 1991;539–566.

Submitted by: Michael Brant-Zawadzki, M.D., F.A.C.R., Hoag Memorial Hospital, Newport Beach, California; Michael Brant-Zawadzki, M.D., F.A.C.R., Senior Editor.

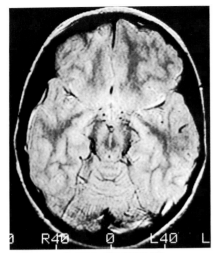

FIG. 73A. SE 2800/30.

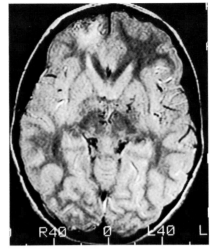

FIG. 73B. SE 2800/30.

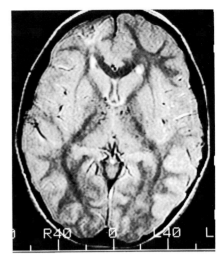

FIG. 73C. SE 2800/30.

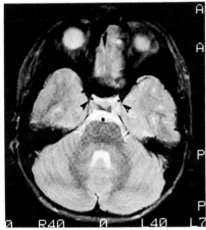

FIG. 73D. SE 2800/80.

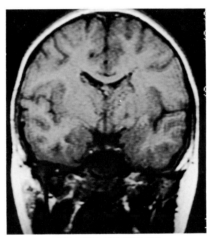

FIG. 73E. SE 500/20.

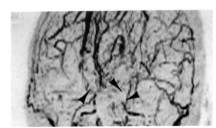

FIG. 73F. 2D TOF MRA (501/9).

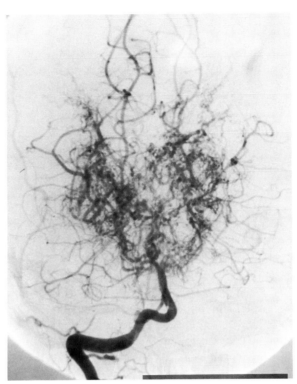

FIG. 73G. Conventional right vertebral artery angiogram.

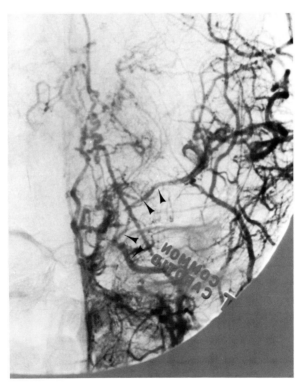

FIG. 73H. Conventional left common carotid artery angiogram.

Clinical History

An 8-year-old female with recurrent strokes.

Findings

Axial proton density images (Figs. 73A–C) show bilaterally prominent vascular signal void in the basal ganglia with right frontal region hyperintense signal from ischemic change. Axial T2-weighted image shows bilateral diminutive cavernous internal carotid arteries (Fig. 73D, *arrowheads*). Basilar artery has normal flow void and lumen caliber. Coronal T1-weighted image (Fig. 73E) further demonstrates enlarged basal ganglia-perforating lenticulostriate arteries. The 2D time-of-flight (TOF) magnetic resonance angiography (MRA) 3D reprojection shows lack of flow-related enhancement (FRE) in both supraclinoid internal carotid arteries (ICA) and M1 segments (Fig. 73F, *arrowheads*) suggesting occlusion. Left common carotid artery (CCA) angiogram shows these vessels lacking FRE are patent but narrowed (Figs. 73G and H, *arrowheads*). Right vertebral artery angiogram demonstrates "puff of cloud" appearance of these vessels.

Diagnosis

Moyamoya disease.

Discussion

The utility of spin-echo MRI in demonstrating narrowed arteries and prominent lenticulostriate and basal ganglia collaterals in moyamoya has been reported (1,2). A limitation of 2D TOF MRA in the imaging of moyamoya is its sensitivity to intravoxel dephasing from complex flow in narrowed arteries, causing loss of FRE and the potential pitfall of diagnosing occlusion. Spin-echo imaging gives supplemental information by depicting these vessels as flow voids. The 3D TOF MRA also may not be an optimal vascular imaging technique for demonstrating the collateral vessels due to saturation effects.

References

1. Fajisawa I, Asato R, Nishimura K, et al. Moyamoya disease: MR imaging. *Radiology* 1987;164:103–105.
2. Spritzer CE, Blinder RA. Vascular applications of magnetic resonance imaging. *Magn Reson Q* 1989;5:205–227.

Submitted by: Orest B. Boyko, M.D., Ph.D., Duke University Medical Center, Durham, North Carolina; Michael Brant-Zawadzki, M.D., F.A.C.R., Senior Editor.

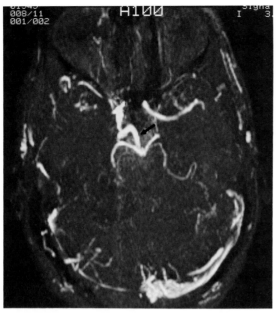

FIG. 74A. 2D TOF MRA collapsed reprojection (45/9/60°).

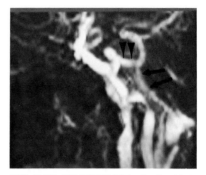

FIG. 74B. 2D TOF MRA stacked lateral reprojection (45/9/60°).

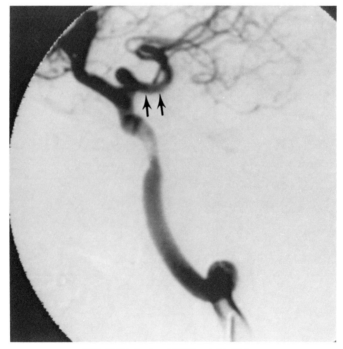

FIG. 74C. Lateral DSA, right ICA.

Clinical History

A 27-year-old male presents for workup of a base of skull tumor.

Findings

On 2D time-of-flight (TOF) magnetic resonance angiography (MRA) an intrasellar arterial anastomosis between the cavernous portion of the right internal carotid artery (ICA) and the basilar artery is identified on 2D collapsed (Fig. 74A, *arrow*) and 3D stacked lateral repro-jection images (Fig. 74B, *arrowheads*). Lateral right ICA digital subtraction angiogram (DSA) (Fig. 74C, *arrows*) confirms the arterial anastomosis. Note proximal basilar artery hypoplasia on the 2D TOF MRA (Fig. 74B, *arrows*).

Diagnosis

Persistent primitive trigeminal artery (PPTA) demonstrated on MRA.

Discussion

PPTA is the most common of the primitive anastomotic vessels and has a reported angiographic incidence of 0.6% (1). In 50% of cases the PPTA penetrates the sella turcica, perforates the dura near the clivus, and joins the basilar artery. In other cases, the artery runs lateral to the sella. The basilar artery proximal to the area of PPTA anastomosis is usually hypoplastic (2). Coexistence of a cerebral aneurysm is reported to be 14% (3), rarely in-volving the PPTA itself. Embryologically the trigeminal artery supplies the two longitudinal neural arteries, which later fuse to form the basilar artery. Failure of the trigeminal artery to involute by 46 days gestation or by the 11.5-mm embryonic stage results in its persistence.

The association of PPTA with any specific disorders of the nervous system is controversial.

References

1. Fields WS. The significance of persistent trigeminal artery: carotid-basilar anastomosis. *Radiology* 1968;91:1096–1101.
2. Fortner AA, Smoker WRK. Persistent primitive trigeminal artery aneurysm evaluated by MR imaging and angiography. *J Comput Assist Tomogr* 1988;12:847–850.
3. George AE, Lin JP, Morantz RA. Intracranial aneurysm of a persistent trigeminal artery. *J Neurosurg* 1971;35:601–604.

Submitted by: Orest B. Boyko, M.D., Ph.D., Duke University Medical Center, Durham, North Carolina; Michael Brant-Zawadzki, M.D., F.A.C.R., Senior Editor.

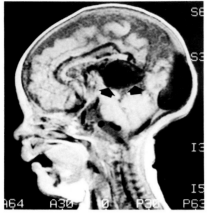

FIG. 75A. Sagittal SE 600/12.

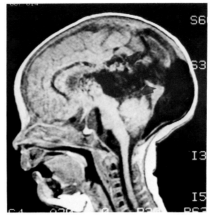

FIG. 75B. Sagittal SE 600/12.

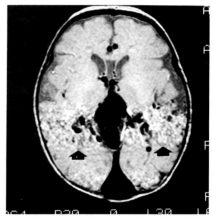

FIG. 75C. Axial SE 2000/32.

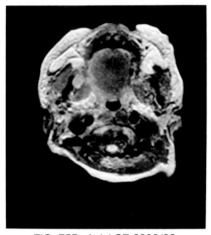

FIG. 75D. Axial SE 2000/32.

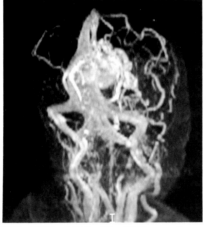

FIG. 75E. MRA 2D TOF gradient-refocused, 45/9.

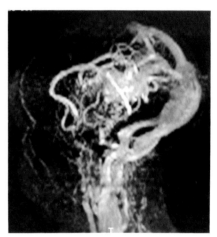

FIG. 75F. MRA 2D TOF gradient-refocused, 45/9.

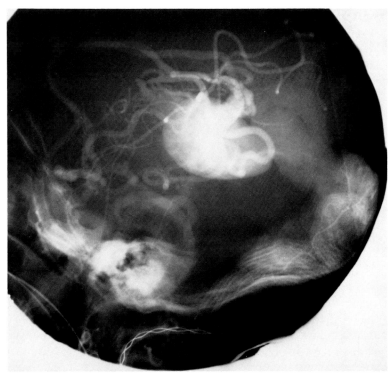

FIG. 75G. Conventional angiogram.

Clinical History

A 4-day-old female with congestive heart failure (CHF).

Findings

Sagittal T1-weighted image (Fig. 75A) demonstrates markedly enlarged vertebral, internal carotid, and anterior cerebral arteries with a vein of Galen malformation (varix) (Figs. 75A and B, *arrowheads*). Venous outflow is into an associated prominent torcular confluence. Axial T2-weighted image reveals flow artifact in the phase-encoding direction (Fig. 75C, *arrowheads*) secondary to pulsatile/turbulent/fast flow in the varix. Axial T2-weighted image in the cervical region shows prominent jugular veins bilaterally (Fig. 75D, *arrowheads*).

The 2D time-of-flight (TOF) magnetic resonance angiography (MRA) reveals in the anteroposterior (Fig. 75E) and lateral (Fig. 75F) projection the venous varix and prominent venous outflow and enlarged feeding arteries seen also on a lateral conventional angiogram in the arterial phase (Fig. 75G) of a left common carotid artery (CCA) injection. On the MRA flow-related enhancement is not present in the most anterior portion of the superior sagittal sinus.

Diagnosis

Vein of Galen malformation (VGM).

Discussion

Vein of Galen malformation describes a heterogeneous patient group with a congenital anomaly of enlarged deep venous structures because of direct arteriovenous fistulas (AVF) to the wall of the vein of Galen (this case) or a complex pial arteriovenous malformation (AVM) draining into the deep venous system. Almost all cases are associated with a venous outflow restriction. The AVF group tends to be younger (mean age 15.3 months) (1). CHF rather than hydrocephalus (not present in this case) tends to be a clinical association in the AVF group. The hydrocephalus can occur because of increased intracranial venous pressure and impaired cerebrospinal fluid reabsorption. Congenital absence of the straight sinus but development of a prominent falcine sinus or inferior sagittal sinus is not uncommon.

MR is superior to CT in the clinical evaluation of VGM except for the detection of calcium.

References

1. Seidenwurm D, Berenstein A, Hyman A, et al. Vein of Galen malformations: correlation of clinical presentation, arteriography, and MR imaging. *AJNR* 1991;12:347–354.
2. Litvak J, Yahr MD, Ransohoff J. Aneurysms of the great vein of Galen and midline cerebral arterio-venous anomalies. *J Neurosurg* 1960;17:945–954.
3. Martelli A, Scotti G, Harwood-Nash DC, et al. Aneurysms of the vein of Galen in children: CT and angiographic correlation. *Neuroradiology* 1980;20:123–133.
4. Quisling RG, Mickle JP. Venous pressure measurements in vein of Galen aneurysms. *AJNR* 1987;10:411–417.

Submitted by: Orest B. Boyko, M.D., Ph.D., Duke University Medical Center, Durham, North Carolina; Michael Brant-Zawadzki, M.D., F.A.C.R., Senior Editor.

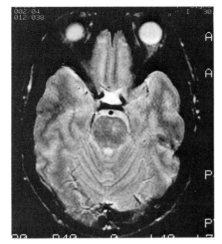

FIG. 76A. SE 2000/80.

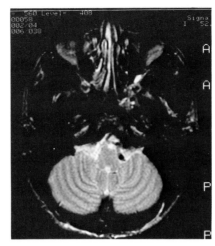

FIG. 76B. SE 2000/80.

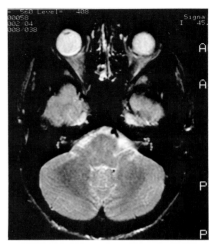

FIG. 76C. SE 2000/80.

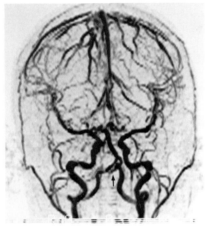

FIG. 76D. 2D TOF MRA.

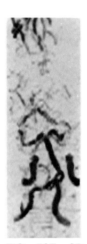

FIG. 76E. 2D TOF MRA.

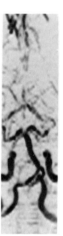

FIG. 76F. 2D TOF MRA.

Clinical History

A 17-year-old male with past history of left cervical vertebral artery pseudoaneurysm and thromboembolism treated by previous balloon occlusion therapy.

Findings

Axial T2-weighted image shows very small old left pontine infarct with normal basilar artery flow void (Fig. 76A). At the foramen magnum (Fig. 76B) both vertebral arteries are unremarkable. On the next anatomic slice (Fig. 76C) the basilar artery has a circular appearance, better visualized on 2D time-of-flight (TOF) magnetic resonance angiography (MRA) (Fig. 76D, *arrow*). Further different masked reprojections demonstrate the unusual configuration of the basilar artery (Figs. 76E and F). Conventional digital subtraction angiogram of the left vertebral artery confirms the MRA findings (Fig. 76G).

Diagnosis

Congenital fenestration of the basilar artery.

Discussion

Fenestration of an artery can be mistaken for aneurysmal dilation because of the angiographic summation of two lumina. The basilar artery is the most common site for fenestration.

Reference

1. Wollschlaeger G, Wollschlaeger PB. In: Newton TH, Potts GA, eds. *The circle of Willis in radiology of the skull and brain.* MediBooks, St. Louis, MO, 1981;1171–1199.

Submitted by: Orest B. Boyko, M.D., Ph.D., Duke University Medical Center, Durham, North Carolina; Michael Brant-Zawadzki, M.D., F.A.C.R., Senior Editor.

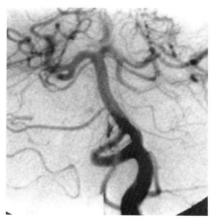

FIG. 76G. Left vertebral artery angiogram.

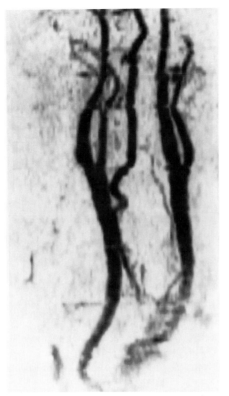

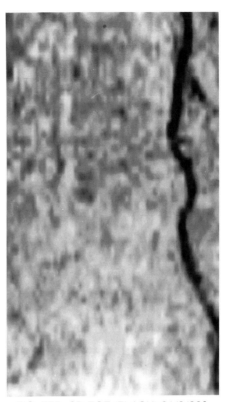

FIG. 77A. 2D TOF (FLASH) 31/9/30°.   FIG. 77B. 2D TOF (FLASH) 31/9/30°.

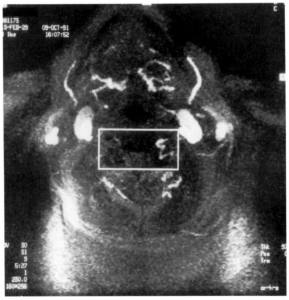

FIG. 77C. Collapsed MRA image.

Clinical History

A 71-year-old male with left arm weakness during heavy work.

Findings

MR angiogram (Fig. 77A) demonstrates unremarkable carotid artery bifurcations with visualization of only the right vertebral artery. However, the study was done with a traveling saturation pulse placed superior to the slice. Subsequent study (Fig. 77B) demonstrates flow of the left vertebral artery when the saturation pulse was placed inferior to the slice.

Diagnosis

Left subclavian steal with retrograde flow in left vertebral artery.

Discussion

Vertebral artery "steal" simply represents a collateralization of distal left subclavian artery flow, when a stenotic lesion occurs proximal to the origin of the vertebral artery. It may become symptomatic, particularly when other causes of poor circulation to the posterior fossa exist. It must be remembered that saturation pulses act to diminish inflow from vessels prior to entering the imaging plane. Thus when vertebral steal is suspected, the saturation band needs to be placed inferior to the imaging slice in order to visualize retrograde arterial flow. Phase contrast angiography could also accomplish this. Note that venous flow is not seen on Fig. 77B; this is due to the selected maximum intensity pixel (MIP) region of interest seen on the collapsed view (Fig. 77C).

References

1. Kadir S. Arteriography of the upper extremities. In: *Diagnostic angiography.* Philadelphia: WB Saunders, 1986;172–206.
2. Newton TH, Wylie EJ. Collateral circulation associated with occlusion of the proximal subclavian and innominate arteries. *AJR* 1964;91:394–405.
3. Ashby RN, Karras BJ, Cannon AH. Clinical and roentgenographic aspects of the subclavian steal syndrome. *AJR* 1963;90:535–545.

Submitted by: Anton N. Hasso, M.D., F.A.C.R., Loma Linda University School of Medicine, Loma Linda, California; Michael Brant-Zawadzki, M.D., F.A.C.R., Senior Editor.

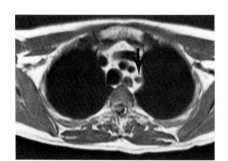

FIG. 78A. SE 2000/20.

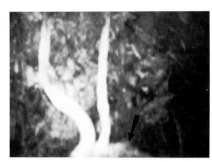

FIG. 78B. 3D TOF MRA, 50/7.

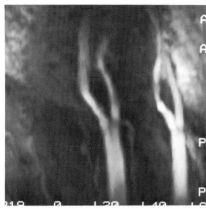

FIG. 78C. 3D TOF MRA, 60/8.

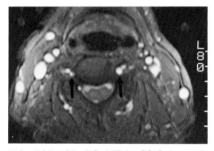

FIG. 78D. 2D PC MRA, 26/9 (magnitude image).

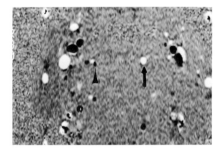

FIG. 78E. 2D PC MRA, 26/9 (phase image).

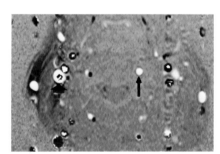

FIG. 78F. 2D PC MRA, 24/10 (phase image).

Clinical History

A 64-year-old male with left arm paresthesias.

Findings

Axial proton density image (Fig. 78A, *arrow*) shows no flow void in the left subclavian artery (SA). The 3D time-of-flight (TOF) magnetic resonance angiography (MRA) shows the occluded stump of the left SA (Fig. 78B, *arrow*). The 3D TOF MRA of the carotid arteries (Fig. 78C) is normal.

The 2D phase contrast (PC) MRA magnitude image shows flow-related enhancement in both vertebral arteries (Fig. 78D, *arrows*). Phase image (flow-encoded direction is superior/inferior with a velocity encoding of 80 cm/sec) reveals reversal of flow in the dominant left ver-

tebral artery (Fig. 78E, *arrow*) (bright pixels indicating flow in the direction of the flow-encoding gradient, superior to inferior) compared to the right vertebral artery (VA) (Fig. 78E, *arrowhead*).

At a velocity encoding (VENC) of 20 cm/sec, the left VA flow reversal is again seen (Fig. 78F, *arrow*). Note artifactual dark pixels central in the right internal jugular vein (Fig. 78F, *arrowhead*) and bright pixels central in the right internal carotid artery because of aliasing of flow in the vessels due to the use of a lower velocity-encoding setting of 20 cm/sec.

Diagnosis

Atherosclerotic occlusion origin of the left subclavian artery with reversal of flow in the left vertebral artery (subclavian steal).

Discussion

Atherosclerosis is the most common underlying cause for the subclavian steal syndrome (1,2). It is predominantly left-sided. The differential diagnosis includes arteritis, trauma, tumor thrombus/encasement, and surgical interruption.

This case illustrates the benefit of directional information obtained from phase contrast MRA. It also illustrates that depending on the velocity encoding (VENC)

chosen by the operator, aliasing artifacts can occur (Fig. 78F). Aliasing is a phenomenon created because the signal from vessels flowing faster than the velocity encoding are incorrectly represented in an image as having slower speed or as flow in the opposite direction. The peak velocities in a vessel greater than the VENC setting will be aliased and usually this is central in a vessel at the lower VENC of 20 cm/sec.

References

1. Reivich M, Holling E, Roberts B, et al. Reversal of blood flow through the vertebral artery and its effect on cerebral circulation. *N Engl J Med* 1961;265:878–885.
2. Fields WS, Lemak NA. Joint study of extracranial arterial occlusion. VII. Subclavian steal—a review of 168 cases. *JAMA* 1972;222:1139–1143.

Submitted by: Orest B. Boyko, M.D., Ph.D., Duke University Medical Center, Durham, North Carolina; Michael Brant-Zawadzki, M.D., F.A.C.R., Senior Editor.

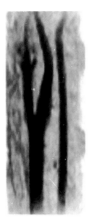
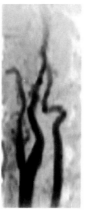
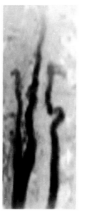
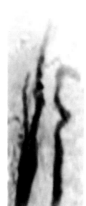
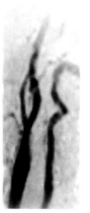
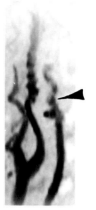
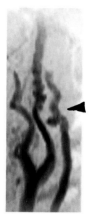

FIG. 79A.
3D TOF
MRA (40/7/
20°).

FIG. 79B.
3D TOF
MRA (40/7/
20°).

FIG. 79C.
3D TOF
MRA (40/7/
20°).

FIG. 79D.
3D TOF
MRA (40/7/
20°).

FIG. 79E.
3D TOF
MRA (40/7/
20°).

FIG. 79F.
3D TOF
MRA (40/7/
20°).

FIG. 79G.
3D TOF
MRA (40/7/
20°).

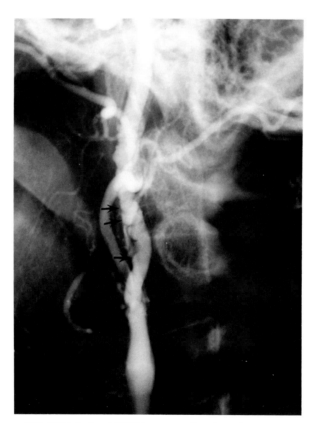

FIG. 79H. Lateral RCCA conventional angiogram.

Clinical History

A 64-year-old female with asymptomatic right carotid bruit.

Findings

The 3D time-of-flight (TOF) magnetic resonance angiography (MRA) 3D reprojection using 0.7 mm thin axial partition images showed no atherosclerotic disease of the right carotid bruit (Fig. 79A). More cephalad imaging using 1.5 mm axial partition images demonstrates on four 3D reprojections (Figs. 79B–E) narrowing and widening of the right internal carotid artery (ICA).

The 3D TOF MRA 3D reprojections (Figs. 79F and G) of the left ICA demonstrates a long segmental narrowing of the proximal left ICA with a string-of-beads appearance. Irregularity of the left vertebral artery is also seen (Fig. 79F, G, *arrowheads*). Right common carotid conventional angiogram verifies the diagnosis (Fig. 79H).

Diagnosis

Fibromuscular dysplasia (FMD).

Discussion

FMD is oftentimes an incidental finding in middle-aged or older women (1). FMD mainly affects the cervical portion of the ICA distal to the carotid bulb. In 75% of cases involvement is bilateral, and the vertebral artery is involved in 15%. Luminal stenosis greater than 60% can occur causing hemodynamic symptoms as well as dissection. There is an increased association of intracranial saccular aneurysm in 20% to 40% of cases.

Reference

1. Houser OW, Baker HL, Sandok BA, et al. Cephalic arterial fibromuscular dysplasia. *Radiology* 1971;101:605.

Submitted by: John Karis, M.D., and Orest B. Boyko, M.D., Ph.D., Duke University Medical Center, Durham, North Carolina; Michael Brant-Zawadzki, M.D., F.A.C.R., Senior Editor.

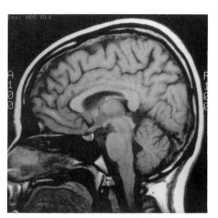
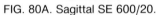

FIG. 80A. Sagittal SE 600/20.

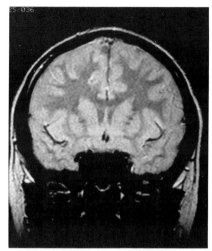

FIG. 80B. Coronal SE 2800/30.

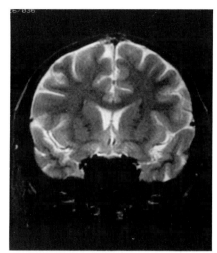

FIG. 80C. Coronal SE 2800/90.

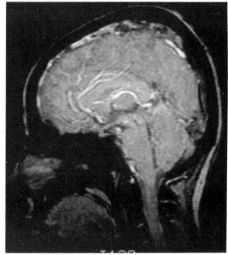

FIG. 80D. 2D GRASS 150/15/50°.

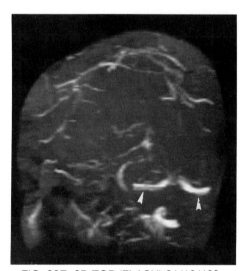

FIG. 80E. 2D TOP (FLASH) 31/10/40°.

Clinical History

A 21-year-old female with headache, vomiting, and papilledema.

Findings

T1-weighted sagittal (Fig. 80A) as well as dual echo coronal (Fig. 80B and C) sequences show no definite abnormality. Note the heterogeneity of signal in the region of the sagittal sinus. A sagittal gradient echo recalled flow sequence (Fig. 80D) was performed, which suggests at least partial occlusion of the superior sagittal sinus. A 2D time-of-flight MR angiogram (Fig. 80E) was performed with saturation of arterial inflow, and with particular attention to the venous phase. This demonstrates to good advantage the occlusion of the sagittal sinus throughout most of its course, with reconstitution of the transverse sinuses (Fig. 80E, *arrowheads*) through cortical veins.

Diagnosis

Sagittal sinus occlusion.

Discussion

In cases where there is no evidence for venous infarction or other parenchymal abnormality, the diagnosis of sagittal sinus occlusion can be quite difficult on conventional MR images. MR angiography with specific venous techniques utilizing a time-of-flight approach, or phase contrast MR angiography with velocity encoding in the venous range can be helpful. The presentation of sagittal sinus occlusion may simply be that of increased intracranial pressure with papilledema. Patients predisposed to this condition are those with hypercoagulable states, dehydration, neoplastic syndromes, as well as those undergoing certain types of chemotherapy.

References

1. Mattle HP, Wentz KU, et al. Cerebral venography with MR. *Radiology* 1991;178:453–458.
2. Tsuruda JS, Shimakawa A, et al. Dural sinus occlusion: evaluation with phase-sensitive gradient-echo MR imaging. *AJNR* 1991;12:481–488.
3. Rippe DJ, Boyko OB, et al. Demonstration of dural sinus occlusion by use of MR angiography. *AJNR* 1990;11:199–201.

Submitted by: Michael Brant-Zawadzki, M.D., F.A.C.R., Hoag Memorial Hospital, Newport Beach, California; Michael Brant-Zawadzki, M.D., F.A.C.R., Senior Editor.

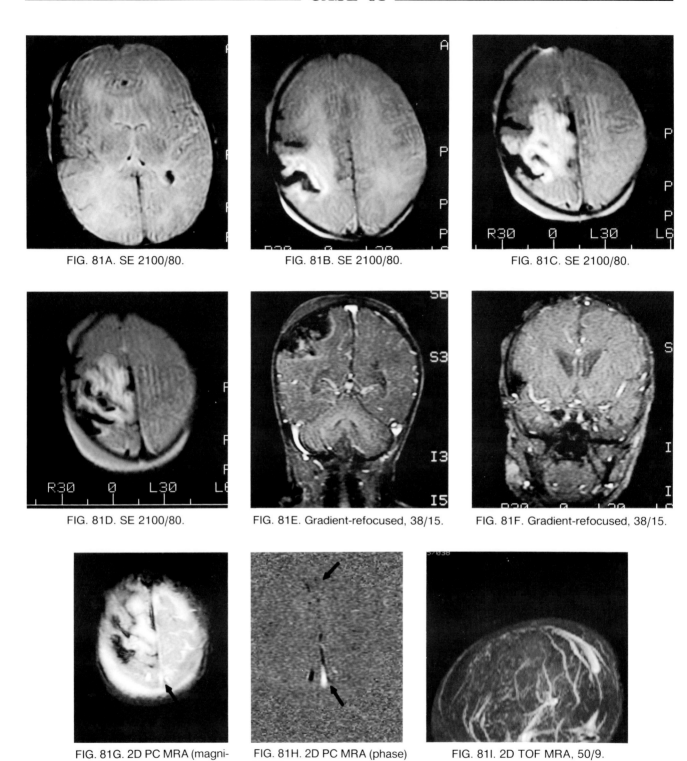

FIG. 81A. SE 2100/80.

FIG. 81B. SE 2100/80.

FIG. 81C. SE 2100/80.

FIG. 81D. SE 2100/80.

FIG. 81E. Gradient-refocused, 38/15.

FIG. 81F. Gradient-refocused, 38/15.

FIG. 81G. 2D PC MRA (magnitude) 26/17.

FIG. 81H. 2D PC MRA (phase) 26/17.

FIG. 81I. 2D TOF MRA, 50/9.

Clinical History

A 35-day-old male infant with seizure.

Findings

Axial T2-weighted image (Fig. 81A) shows left intraventricular hypointense blood clot (deoxyhemoglogin) and higher convexity images (Figs. 81B–D) show blood products (hematoma) in the right cerebral hemisphere. Regions of decreased signal intensity (Fig. 81D) could represent lack of signal from flow void or local magnetic field inhomogeneity from blood products (deoxyhemoglobin). Both anterior and posterior superior sagittal sinus (SSS) (Fig. 81D) demonstrate hypointense signal, suggesting patency and flow void.

Gradient-refocused coronal image (Fig. 81E) demonstrates bright signal of flow [flow-related enhancement (FRE)] of the posterior SSS. The major component of the right cerebral lesion shows no FRE, indicating that the areas of decreased signal on T2-weighted images (Figs. 81B–D) were not flow void vessels but blood clot. More anterior image (Fig. 81F) shows *no* FRE of the anterior SSS, indicating the presence of venous thrombosis. The apparent flow void of the anterior SSS on SE images (Figs. 81B–D) is secondary to loss of signal from deoxyhemoglobin in thrombus, mimicking flow void.

The 2D phase contrast (PC) magnetic resonance angiography (MRA) reveals (with corresponding magnitude) bright FRE of the patent posterior SSS and the lack of FRE in the anterior SSS (Figs. 81G and H, *arrowheads*). A velocity encoding of 20 cm/sec was used. The 2D time-of-flight (TOF) MRA demonstrates on 3D reprojection image (Fig. 81I) the patent posterior SSS and the lack of FRE of the anterior SSS and the lack of anterior cortical veins draining into the superior sagittal sinus.

Diagnosis

Anterior SSS thrombosis with right cerebral hemispheric venous infarct.

Discussion

Methemoglobin can have high signal intensity on spin-echo and gradient-refocused images, mimicking flow (1). Utilization of phase MRA (2,3) can allow for distinguishing hyperintense thrombus on gradient-refocused images (2,3) as illustrated by this case in the right cerebral hemisphere. MRA provides further supplemental information by eliminating the potential pitfall of hypointense signal of deoxyhemoglobin, mimicking flow-void on spin-echo imaging. PC MRA offers the ability for generating magnitude and phase images during the same acquisition time (3).

TOF MRA is proving reliable to demonstrate major venous sinuses (1). Although absence of a vein or sinus on MRA raises the possibility of occlusion, the spin-echo images can be used to exclude an anatomical absence of the sinus as accounting for the absence of FRE on MRA images.

References

1. Mattle HP, Wentz KU, Edelman RR, et al. Cerebral venography with MR. *Radiology* 1991;178:453–458.
2. Nadel L, Braun IF, Kraftka, et al. Intracranial vascular abnormalities: value of MR phase imaging to distinguish thrombus from flowing blood. *AJNR* 1991;11:1133–1140.
3. Tsuruda JS, Shimakawa A, Pelc NJ, et al. Dural sinus occlusion: evaluation with phase-sensitive gradient-echo MR imaging. *AJNR* 1991;12:481–488.

Submitted by: Orest B. Boyko, M.D., Ph.D., Duke University Medical Center, Durham, North Carolina; Michael Brant-Zawadzki, M.D., F.A.C.R., Senior Editor.

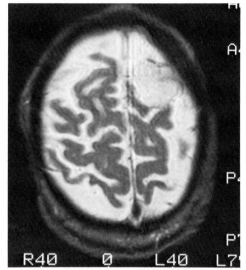

FIG. 82A. SE 3200/80.

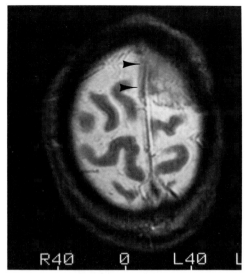

FIG. 82B. SE 3200/80.

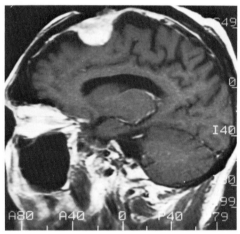

FIG. 82C. Contrast 500/20.

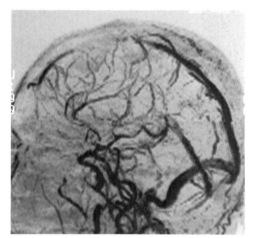

FIG. 82D. 2D TOF MRA, 50/9.

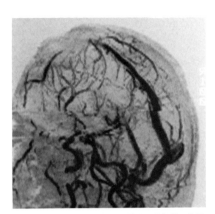

FIG. 82E. 2D TOF MRA, 50/9. 3-D stacked reprojection.

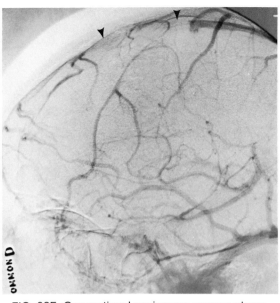

FIG. 82F. Conventional angiogram, venous phase.

Clinical History

A 61-year-old male with long-standing history of erosive calvarial lesion.

Findings

T2-weighted axial images (Figs. 82A and B) show an extraaxial lesion in the high convexity left frontal lobe. High convexity image suggests infiltration into the anterior superior sagittal sinus (SSS) (Fig. 82B, *arrowheads*). Contrast-enhanced T1-weighted sagittal image (Fig. 82C) better delineates the extraaxial mass with homogeneous enhancement of the SSS subjacent to the mass and posteriorly. The calvarium and scalp is eroded in the region overlying the mass. Normal flow void indicating patency of the superior sagittal sinus is seen posteriorly. The 2D time-of-flight MR angiograms (MRA) of the right cerebral hemisphere on stacked 3D reprojection images (Figs. 82D and E) show lack of flow in the anterior portion of the superior sagittal sinus overlying the mass. Conventional angiogram also demonstrates thrombosis of the anterior portion of the superior sagittal sinus (Fig. 82F, *arrowheads*).

Diagnosis

Sagittal sinus thrombosis due to invasion by meningioma.

Discussion

High-field MR imaging to diagnose cerebral venous thrombosis has been shown to be useful (1). This case illustrates that when tumor directly invades a venous sinus it does not yield the same signal intensity parameters as expected of bland thrombus. Although the flow void can be clearly seen in the posterior superior sagittal sinus, the lack of coronal T2-weighted sequences makes diagnosis regarding flow void in the anterior sinus difficult. Contrast enhancement may not be helpful since tumor thrombus within the sinus can enhance and slow flow in venus sinuses can also mimic enhancement. In this case MRA clearly defines the lack of flow in the anterior superior sinus confirmed by the gold standard conventional angiogram. The 3D stacked images were postprocessed to reflect only the venous anatomy of the right cerebral hemisphere including the superior sagittal sinus. The role of MRA in cerebral venous thrombosis is currently being defined (2–4).

References

1. Macchi PJ, Grossman RI, Gomori JM, et al. High field MR imaging of cerebral venous thrombosis. *J Comput Assist Tomogr* 1986;10:10–15.
2. Rippe DJ, Boyko OB, Spritzer CE, et al. Demonstration of dural sinus occlusion by use of MR angiography. *AJNR* 1990;11:199–201.
3. Mattle HP, Wentz KU, Edelman RR, et al. Cerebral venography with MR. *Radiology* 1991;178:453–458.
4. Tsuruda JS, Shimakawa A, Pelc NJ, et al. Dural sinus occlusion: evaluation with phase-sensitive gradient-echo MR imaging. *AJNR* 1991;12:481–488.

Submitted by: Orest B. Boyko, M.D., Ph.D., Duke University Medical Center, Durham, North Carolina; Michael Brant-Zawadzki, M.D., F.A.C.R., Senior Editor.

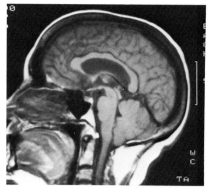

FIG. 83A. SE 600/20.

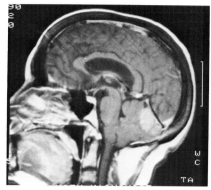

FIG. 83B. Contrast SE 600/20.

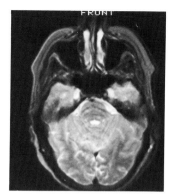

FIG. 83C. SE 2400/90.

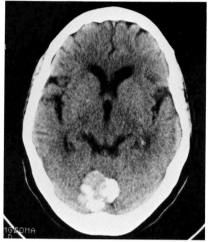

FIG. 83D. CT.

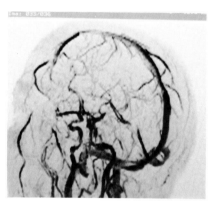

FIG. 83E. 2D TOF MRA, 45/9.

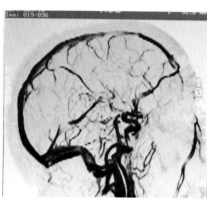

FIG. 83F. 2D TOF MRA, 45/9.

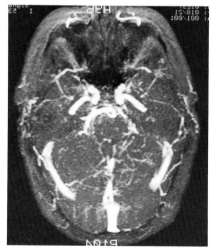

FIG. 83G. 2D TOF MRA, 45/9.

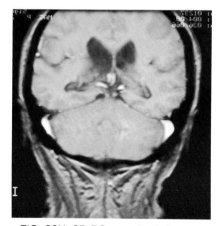

FIG. 83H. 2D PC magnitude image.

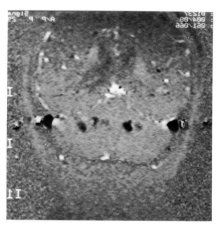

FIG. 83I. 2D PC phase image.

Clinical History

A 64-year-old female with headache.

Findings

Sagittal T1-weighted image shows a dural-based isointense mass with brain (Fig. 83A). Normal flow void in the vein of Galen and straight sinus (Fig. 83B) is shown following gadolinium (Gd)-DTPA injection (Fig. 83A). T2-weighted image poorly defines the mass (Fig. 83C). CT scan without contrast reveals the mass to be calcified (Fig. 83D). The 2D time-of-flight (TOF) magnetic resonance angiography (MRA) in a 3D reprojection shows normal flow-related enhancement (FRE) of the internal cerebral veins bilaterally and the straight sinus (Fig. 83E) but discordant lack of flow-related enhancement (FRE) (Fig. 83F) at the junction of the vein of Galen and straight sinus. The 2D TOF MRA 2D collapsed reprojection demonstrates continuity of FRE (Fig. 83G) in this region.

Diagnosis

Calcified tentorial meningioma with venous sinus patency.

Discussion

Detection of calcium on spin-echo imaging can be difficult. This case illustrates that MRA findings should always be correlated with the flow phenomena observed on spin-echo images.

The lack of visualized FRE at the junction of the vein of Galen and straight sinus suggesting occlusion cannot be confirmed on the sagittal T1-weighted images showing normal flow void. This artifact on MRA is partially caused by loss of signal due to in-plane flow on the axial partition images and artifact of signal dropout by the reprojection algorithm [maximum intensity pixel (MIP)] (1). All the 2D collapsed reprojections show all flow superimposed together, thus falsely "connecting" the midline vein of Galen and straight sinus structures.

Imaging perpendicular to flowing vessels maximizes the FRE signal as seen on 2D phase contrast (PC) MRA partitions, where both magnitude (Fig. 83H) and phase images sensitive to flow in the anterior-posterior direction (Fig. 83I) show bright signal and normal flow direction at the vein of Galen (2).

References

1. Anderson CM, Saloner D, Tsuruda JS, et al. Artifacts in maximum-intensity-projection display of MR angiograms. *AJR* 1990;154:623–629.
2. Tsuruda JS, Shimakawa A, Pelc NJ, Saloner D. Dural sinus occlusion: evaluation with phase-sensitive gradient-echo MR imaging. *AJNR* 1991;12:481–488.

Submitted by: Orest B. Boyko, M.D., Ph.D., Duke University Medical Center, Durham, North Carolina; Michael Brant-Zawadzki, M.D., F.A.C.R., Senior Editor.

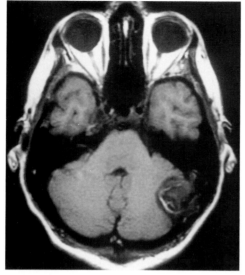

FIG. 84A. Axial SE 2800/90.

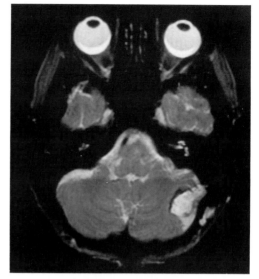

FIG. 84B. Axial SE 600/20.

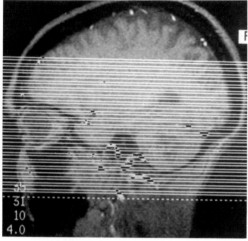

FIG. 84C. Graphic prescription.

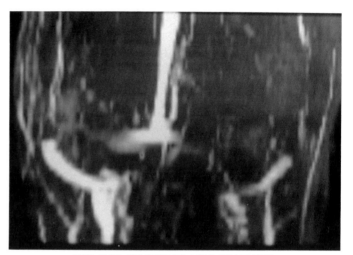

FIG. 84D. 2D TOF (FLASH) 36/10/40°.

Clinical History

A 58-year-old female with left-sided hearing loss.

Findings

A tumor mass is seen involving the left retromastoid calvarium, in fact eroding through it (Figs. 84A and B). The question of transverse sigmoid sinus occlusion arose prior to surgical exploration.

An MR angiogram with 2D axial partition acquisition and saturation of arterial inflow suggests complete occlusion of the left transverse sinus (Fig. 84C and D). However, a coronal 2D partition acquisition (Fig. 84E and F) shows that there is a focal area of stenosis in the proximal left transverse sinus; however, the distal left transverse and sigmoid sinus at the level of the tumor demonstrates patency.

Diagnosis

Epidermoid tumor eroding the calvarium but not occluding the left transverse sinus.

Discussion

This study demonstrates the potential for flow signal saturation when the slices are acquired parallel to the plane of flow (in-plane flow). In this case, the slow flow in the left transverse sinus due to the focal stenosis produced saturation of the in-plane flow. However, the coronal orientation placed the flow perpendicular to the slices, thus improving inflow of unsaturated spins, and more accurately delineating the patent nature of the left transverse sinus while excluding the possibility of tumor invasion.

References

1. Mattle HP, Wentz KU, et al. Cerebral venography with MR. *Radiology* 1991;178:453–458.
2. Rippe DJ, Boyko OB, et al. Demonstration of dural sinus occlusion by use of MR angiography. *AJNR* 1990;11:199–201.
3. Lewin JS, Laub G. Intracranial MR angiography: a direct comparison of three time-of-flight techniques. *AJNR* 1991;12:1133–1139.

Submitted by: Michael Brant-Zawadzki, M.D., F.A.C.R., Hoag Memorial Hospital, Newport Beach, California, Michael Brant-Zawadzki, M.D., F.A.C.R., Senior Editor.

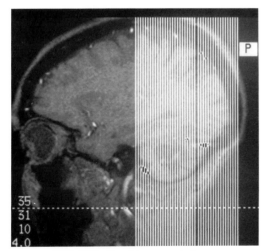

FIG. 84E. Graphic prescription.

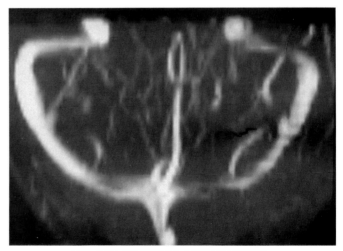

FIG. 84F. 2D TOF (FLASH) 36/10/40°.

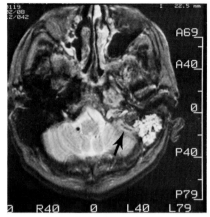

FIG. 85A. SE 3200/80.

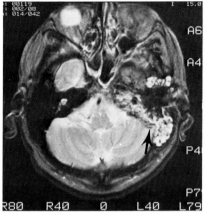

FIG. 85B. SE 500/20.

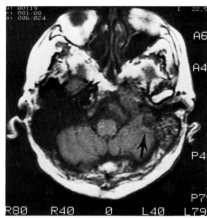

FIG. 85C. SE 3200/80.

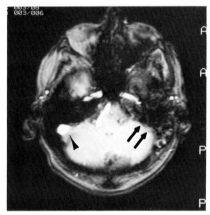

FIG. 85D. 2D PC MRA, 24/13 (magnitude image).

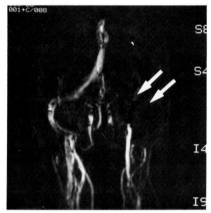

FIG. 85E. 2D PC MRA, 29/15 (slab speed image).

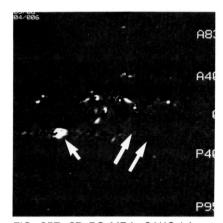

FIG. 85F. 2D PC MRA, 24/13 (phase image).

Clinical History

A 59-year-old male with left ear pain.

Findings

Axial T2-weighted images show signal in the left transverse/sigmoid venous sinus complex (Fig. 85A and B; *arrow*), which is isointense to brain on T1-weighted images (Fig. 85C). Note signal intensity and lack of aeration of the left mastoid air cells (Fig. 85A–C).

The 2D phase contrast (PC) magnetic resonance angiography (MRA) shows flow-related enhancement (FRE) in the right transverse/sigmoid venous sinus on the magnitude image (Fig. 85D, *arrowhead*), but not the left. The 2D PC MRA slab technique in an anteroposterior projection shows lack of flow in the left transverse/sigmoid sinus (Fig. 85E, *arrows*).

Diagnosis

Left transverse/sigmoid venous sinus thrombosis secondary to mastoiditis.

Discussion

MRA is proving to be an adjunct to MR imaging of sinus thrombosis (1,2). In the era of antibiotics, venous sinus thrombophlebitis is uncommon (3). As this case illustrates, the value of the phase image is in the ability to subtract out signal from stationary protons such as clot, mastoid fluid, or bone, and highlight the presence of signal from flowing spins at the base of the skull. The phase image can be obtained individually (Fig. 85F), and in this case demonstrates flow-related enhancement in the right sigmoid sinus (*arrowhead*), but not the left (*arrows*).

References

1. Nadel L, Braun IF, Kraft KA, et al. MRI of intracranial sinovenous thrombosis: the role of phase imaging. *Magn Reson Imaging* 1990;8:315–318.
2. Tsuruda JS, Shimakawa A, Pelc NJ, et al. Dural sinus occlusion: evaluation with phase-sensitive gradient-echo MR imaging. *AJNR* 1991;12:481–488.
3. Southwick FS, Richardson EP, Swartz MN. Septic thrombosis of the dural venous sinuses. *Medicine* 1986;65:82–106.

Submitted by: Orest B. Boyko, M.D., Ph.D., Duke University Medical Center, Durham, North Carolina; Michael Brant-Zawadzki, M.D., F.A.C.R., Senior Editor.

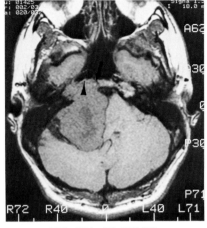

FIG. 86A. SE 500/20.

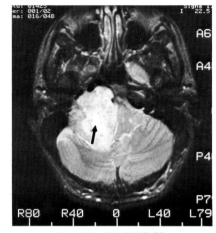

FIG. 86B. SE 2500/80.

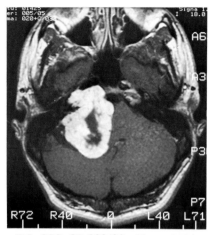

FIG. 86C. SE 600/20 with contrast.

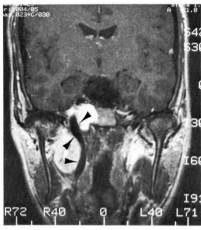

FIG. 86D. SE 383/20 with contrast.

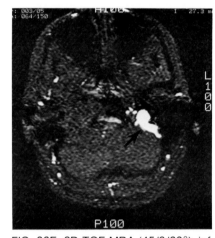

FIG. 86E. 2D TOF MRA (45/9/60°), inf sat pulse.

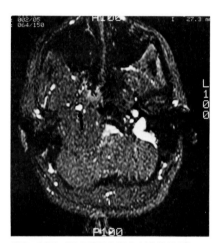

FIG. 86F. 2D TOF MRA (45/9/60°), no sat pulse.

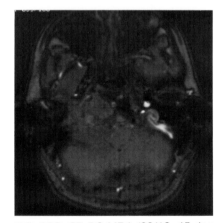

FIG. 86G. 2D PC MRA (28/12; 45 deg flip angle; VENC 10, magnitude image.

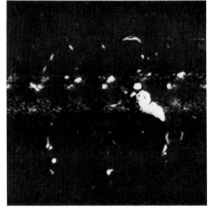

FIG. 86H. 2D PC MRA (speed image).

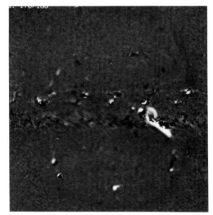

FIG. 86I. 2D PC MRA (phase image; superior/inferior).

Clinical History

A 21-year-old male presents with difficulty in swallowing.

Findings

Axial T1-weighted MR image (Fig. 86A) demonstrates large extraaxial base of skull mass compressing the cerebellum and midbrain. There is erosion of the right medial clivus (Fig. 86A, *arrow*) and petrous apex with encasement and anterior displacement of the petrous portion of an enlarged right internal carotid artery (RICA) (Fig. 86A, *arrowhead*). The lesion has a conspicuous central region of low signal intensity (long T1), which becomes hyperintense on T2-weighted MR imaging (Fig. 86B, *arrow*). This area does not enhance with gadolinium (Gd)-DTPA (Fig. 86C), indicative of a cystic component. Extension of the tumor through the base of the skull with encasement and displacement of the enlarged cervical portion of the RICA (Fig. 86D, *arrowheads*) is demonstrated on coronal T1-weighted images.

The 2D time-of-flight (TOF) magnetic resonance angiography (MRA) using an inferior saturation pulse (ISP) shows flow-related enhancement (FRE) in a prominent left jugular bulb, sigmoid sinus complex (JBSSC) (Fig. 86E, *arrow*) but no FRE in the right JBSSC. Repeat 2D TOF MRA without the ISP again demonstrates no flow in the right JBSSC but the displaced right ICA is now visualized (Fig. 86F, *arrow*).

The 2D phase contrast (PC) magnetic resonance angiography (MRA) shows on magnitude image (Fig. 86G) the tumor mass enlarging the jugular foramen and FRE only in the left JBSSC. The 2D PC MRA speed image (Fig. 86H) depicts the same FRE magnitude information as in Fig. 86G, but the stationary proton signal is subtracted out. The 2D PC MRA phase image sensitive to flow in the superior to inferior direction again depicts only pulsatile artifact and ghosting overlying the right JBSSC originating from the left JBSSC (Fig. 86I). The left JBSSC demonstrates mixed pixel intensity due to aliasing that has occurred at the low velocity encoding used (10 cm/sec) and possible turbulence due to increased outflow on the left because of the obstruction on the right.

Diagnosis

Extraaxial cystic schwannoma with thrombosis of the right JBSSC.

Discussion

Schwannomas of nerves IX, X, and XI are uncommon and can mimic an intraaxial brain stem tumor (1). Enlargement of the jugular foramen is the most common radiographic sign. Although lack of flow void and thrombosis of the right JBSSC could be inferred from spin-echo images in this case, MRA has an evolving role to demonstrate directly venous sinus thrombosis (2).

In this case 2D TOF with and without saturation pulses and 2D PC confirmed right JBSSC thrombosis due to tumor infiltration. The 2D PC MRA may have an advantage over 2D TOF MRA where stationary proton signal on the magnitude image (Fig. 86G) is subtracted out yielding either a speed image (Fig. 86H) (composite image of flow but with no specific directional information) on phase image (Fig. 86I) (computer-generated image yielding directional information relative to a flow-encoding gradient, in this image superior to inferior).

References

1. Sigal R, D'Anthouard F, David P, et al. Cystic schwannoma mimicking a brain stem tumor: MR features. *J Comput Assist Tomogr* 1990;14:662–664.
2. Rippe DJ, Boyko OB, Spritzer CE, et al. Demonstration of dural sinus occlusion by the use of MR angiography. *AJNR* 1990;11:199–201.
3. Turski P, Bernstein M, Boyko OB, et al. *Vascular magnetic resonance imaging.* Milwaukee, WI: GE Medical Systems, 1990.

Submitted by: Orest B. Boyko, M.D., Ph.D., Department of Radiology, Duke University Medical Center, Durham, North Carolina; Michael Brant-Zawadzki, M.D., F.A.C.R., Senior Editor.

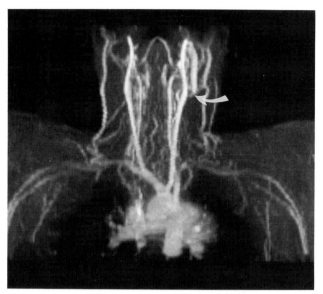
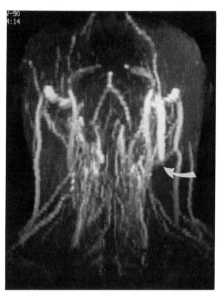

FIG. 87A. 2D TOF (FLASH) 31/10/40°.   FIG. 87B. 2D TOF (FLASH) 31/10/40°.

Clinical History

A 42-year-old female, status post–central line placement in the left jugular vein, now presents with question of venous occlusion.

Findings

The 2D time-of-flight angiographic sequences performed through the neck and upper chest (Fig. 87A and B) shows obvious asymmetry of the jugular veins. The left internal jugular vein fills to the mid-neck level (*arrow*) and internal right jugular vein is not identified.

Diagnosis

Distal left jugular venous occlusion; complete occlusion right internal jugular vein.

Discussion

The capability of MR angiography extends to the venous circulation as well. Jugular venous flow is sufficiently brisk to produce time-of-flight phenomenon and therefore occlusive disease of the venous system can be evaluated. Saturation pulses placed inferiorly at the level of inflowing arteries help diminish superimposition of the arterial system on the venous structures (Fig. 87B).

However, in rapidly flowing vessels, such as the carotid and vertebral arteries, there is sufficient time for the blood to recover its longitudinal magnetization and therefore produce signal distal to the saturation band, as seen in this case. Phase contrast angiography can effectively eliminate the signal from the arterial structures by appropriate choice of velocity encodings.

References

1. Mattle HP, Wentz KU, et al. Cerebral venography with MR. *Radiology* 1991;178:453–458.
2. Edelman RR, Wentz KU, et al. Projection arteriography and venography: initial clinical results with MR. *Radiology* 1989;172:351–357.
3. Felmlee JP, Ehman RL. Spatial presaturation: a method for suppressing flow artefacts and improving depiction of vascular anatomy in MR imaging. *Radiology* 1987;164:559–564.

Submitted by: Michael Brant-Zawadzki, M.D., F.A.C.R., Hoag Memorial Hospital, Newport Beach, California; Michael Brant-Zawadzki, M.D., F.A.C.R., Senior Editor.

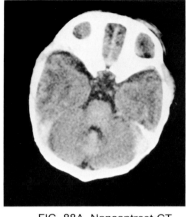

FIG. 88A. Noncontrast CT.

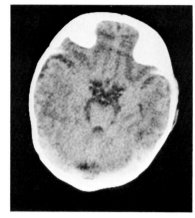

FIG. 88B. Noncontrast CT.

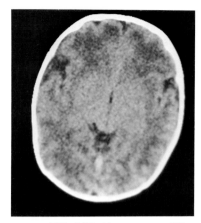

FIG. 88C. Noncontrast CT.

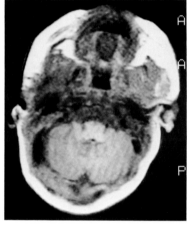

FIG. 88D. SE 500/20.

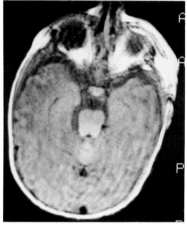

FIG. 88E. SE 500/20.

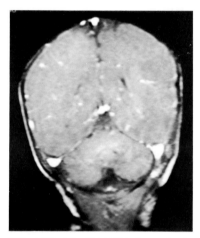

FIG. 88F. 2D PC MRA (magnitude image).

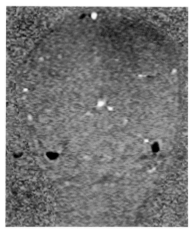

FIG. 88G. 2D PC MRA (phase image).

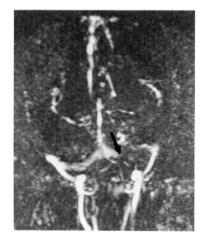

FIG. 88H. 2D PC MRA (speed image).

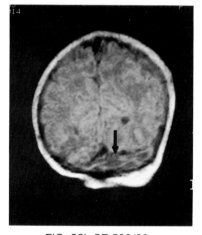

FIG. 88I. SE 500/20.

Clinical History

A 10-month-old with seizure.

Findings

Noncontrast CT scans show hyperdense sigmoid, transverse, and straight venous sinuses (Figs. 88A–C) without venous infarct. Axial T1-weighted image reveals flow void in the venous sinuses (Figs. 88D and E).

The 2D phase contrast (PC) magnetic resonance angiography (MRA) (velocity encoding 20 cm/sec) shows hyperintense signal of flow-related enhancement (FRE) in all the dural venous sinuses (Fig. 88F) with expected symmetry of direction of flow on the corresponding phase image (Fig. 88G). The flow-encoding direction is anterior-posterior (AP), and dark pixels (transverse sinus) indicate flow in the direction opposite to the flow-encoding direction (posterior to anterior).

The 2D PC MRA 2D collapsed postprocessed total flow or speed image (composite image made up of flows in multiple directions with magnitude but no specific direction information) confirms flow in the torcula, transverse, and sigmoid sinuses (Fig. 88H). Note apparent lack of flow distal to the torcula on the left (Fig. 88H, *arrow*) correlating with anatomic hypoplasia of the venous sinus as suggested on coronal T1-weighted image (Fig. 88I, *arrow*).

Diagnosis

Hyperdense venous sinuses without evidence for thrombosis.

Discussion

Hyperdense venous sinuses on CT scans can be a normal finding in children (1,2). This finding can be associated with an elevated hematocrit (or if the sinus is dilated, with an elevated central venous pressure or cardiac failure) (3).

This case illustrates that any lack of FRE (Fig. 88H; *arrow*) on MRA images needs to be correlated with spin-echo images (Fig. 88I; *arrow*) to exclude atretic, hypoplastic, or congenitally absent vessels (4).

References

1. Osborn AG, Anderson RE, Wing SD. The false falx sign. *Radiology* 1980;134:421–425.
2. Segall HD, Ahmadi J, McComb JG, et al. Computed tomographic observations pertinent to intracranial venous thrombotic and occlusive disease in childhood. *Radiology* 1982;143:441–449.
3. Kuharik MA, Edwards MK. Cerebral venous distention associated with cardiac failure in infants. *AJNR* 1987;8:657–659.
4. Mattle HP, Wentz KU, Edelman RR, et al. Cerebral venography with MR. *Radiology* 1991;178:453–458.

Submitted by: Orest B. Boyko, M.D., Ph.D., Duke University Medical Center, Durham, North Carolina; Michael Brant-Zawadzki, M.D., F.A.C.R., Senior Editor.

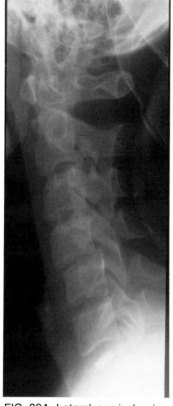

FIG. 89A. Lateral cervical spine radiograph.

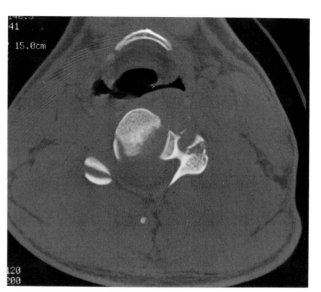

FIG. 89B. Axial CT.

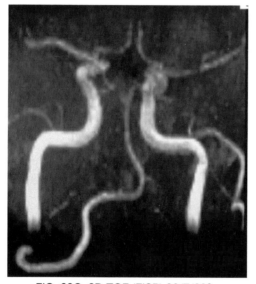

FIG. 89C. 3D TOF (FISP) 30/7/20°.

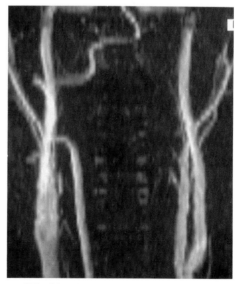

FIG. 89D. 2D TOF (FLASH) 31/9/30°.

Clinical History

A 25-year-old with cervical spine trauma.

212

Findings

The plain x-rays demonstrate subluxation at the C5-6 level (Fig. 89A). The CT scan shows a fracture of the left lateral mass with extension into the foramen transversarium (Fig. 89B). The 3D time-of-flight magnetic resonance angiogram (MRA) at the base of the skull (Fig. 89C) demonstrates only a small stump entering the basilar artery from the left vertebral artery region. A cervical MRA (2D time-of-flight) (Fig. 89D) shows absence of the left vertebral.

Diagnosis

Left vertebral artery occlusion as a result of trauma.

Discussion

This case demonstrates the value of cross-sectional imaging and MR angiography in patient management. In this particular case, the surgeons were planning to stabilize the cervical spine immediately after the trauma. Demonstration of vascular injury lead to more conservative management. An intraarterial angiogram was done to verify the impression of vascular trauma and shows the stump of the left vertebral artery (Fig. 89E, *arrow*) and its reconstitution high in the neck through thyrocervical branches (Fig. 89F, *arrow*). The patient was kept in the cervical collar until follow-up MRA demonstrated reconstitution of the vessel (Fig. 89G). At that point, surgical fusion was performed.

The presence of a large foramen transversarium on the CT rules out congenital hypoplasia as a cause for nonvisualization of the left vertebral artery. The intraarterial angiogram helps to verify this impression.

References

1. Davis JM, Zimmerman RA. Injury of the carotid and vertebral arteries: review article. *Neuroradiology* 1983;25:55–69.
2. Buscaglia LC, Crowhurst HD. Vertebral artery trauma. *Am J Surg* 1979;138:269–279.
3. Schneider RC, Bosch EC, et al. Blood vessel trauma following head and neck injuries. *Clin Neurosurg* 1972;19:312–354.

Submitted by: Michael Brant-Zawadzki, M.D., F.A.C.R., Hoag Memorial Hospital, Newport Beach, California; Michael Brant-Zawadzki, M.D., F.A.C.R., Senior Editor.

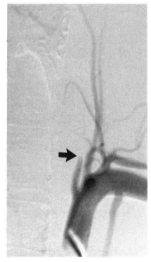

FIG. 89E. Intraarterial angiogram DSA LSA.

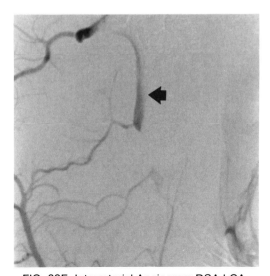

FIG. 89F. Intraarterial Angiogram DSA LCA.

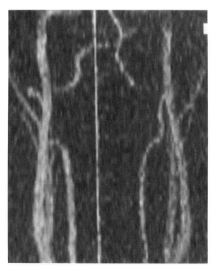

FIG. 89G. 2D TOF (FLASH) 31/9/30°.

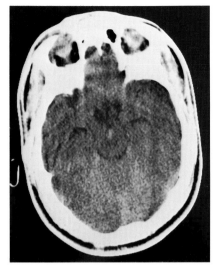

FIG. 90A. Noncontrast CT.

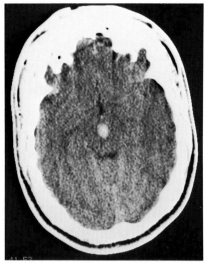

FIG. 90B. Noncontrast CT.

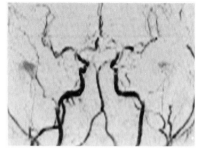

FIG. 90C. 2D TOF MRA anterior posterior view (55/9/60° flip angle).

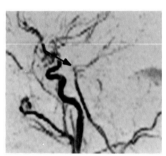

FIG. 90D. 2D TOF MRA Lateral view (55/9/60°).

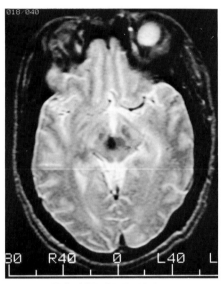

FIG. 90E. SE 2100/80.

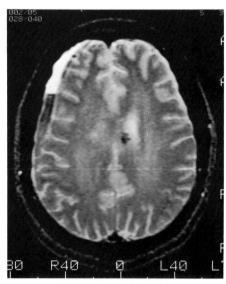

FIG. 90F. SE 2100/80.

Clinical History

A 22-year-old male presents with altered mental status after a motor vehicle accident.

214

Findings

CT scan images show an anterior midline brain stem hemorrhage (Figs. 90A and B). A question of a basilar tip aneurysm arose. The 2D time-of-flight (TOF) magnetic resonance angiography (MRA) in the anteroposterior (Fig. 90C) and the lateral (Fig. 90D) projection demonstrate a normal tip of the basilar artery (Fig. 90D, *arrow*).

T2-weighted images 10 weeks later show hypointense midbrain signal of hemosiderin from the resorbed clot (Fig. 90E) and hemosiderin in the corpus callosum (Fig. 90F) from shear injury. Note the incidental right frontal subdural (Fig. 90F).

Diagnosis

Traumatic brain stem hemorrhage from blunt head trauma.

Discussion

Brain stem hematoma associated with trauma occurs in 0.75% to 3.6% of closed head trauma patients. The midline anterior brain stem, as in this case, is the most frequent site, 69% (1). The survival rate can be as high as 71% (1). Craniocaudal displacement of the brain places stress on the penetrating vessels in the anterior brain stem since the basilar and proximal posterior cerebral vessels are tethered to the skull base through their connections to the cerebral vessels. Rotational shear injuries result in injury to the dorsolateral region of the rostral brain stem.

Reference

1. Meyer CA, Mirvis SE, Wolf AL, et al. Acute traumatic midbrain hemorrhage: experimental and clinical observations with CT. *Radiology* 1991;179:813–818.

Submitted by: Orest B. Boyko, M.D., Ph.D., Duke University Medical Center, Durham, North Carolina; Michael Brant-Zawadzki, M.D., F.A.C.R., Senior Editor.

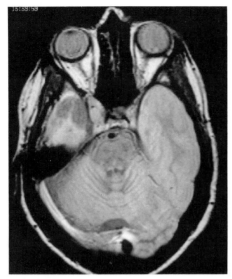 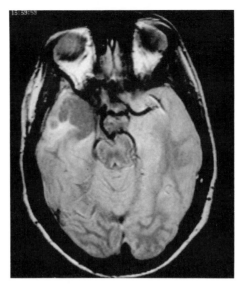

FIG. 91A. Axial SE 2800/22.

FIG. 91B. Axial SE 2800/22.

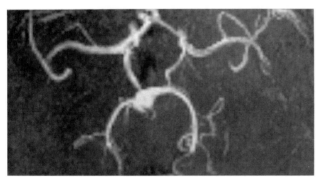 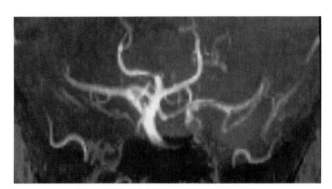

FIG. 91C. 3D TOF (FISP) 35/7/25°.

FIG. 91D. 3D TOF (FISP) 35/7/25°.

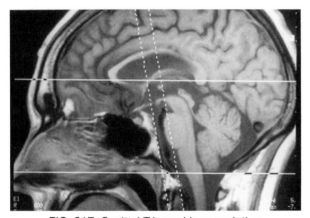 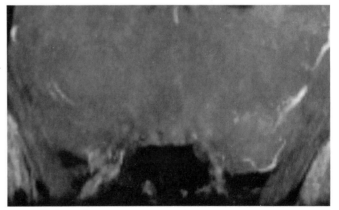

FIG. 91E. Sagittal T1 graphic prescription.

FIG. 91F. 3D TOF (FISP) coronal projection 35/7/25°.

Clinical History

An 18-year-old male with history of right cavernous-carotid fistula and iatrogenic bilateral occlusions of both carotid arteries. The current study was performed to evaluate the intracranial circulation.

Findings

The absence of normal flow void in both carotid arteries is shown on the conventional MR first echo image of the long TR sequence (Fig. 91A). The adjacent slice demonstrates prominent flow void in the right posterior communicating artery (Fig. 91B), as well as in the tip of the right internal carotid and left middle cerebral artery systems. The MR angiographic study (Fig. 91C) demonstrates patency of the circle of Willis with filling of the basilar, posterior cerebral, posterior communicating, and middle cerebral artery complexes throughout. Note the absence of carotid artery filling below the clinoid level and also the basilar and right posterior communicating artery enlargement (Fig. 91D).

Using saturation pulses (Fig. 91E, *dotted lines*), one can verify the importance of the basilar artery as the single source of inflow to the brain. The *solid lines* in Fig. 91E represent the 3D axial slab location. Utilizing this technique, any flow signal through the basilar artery to the brain will be eliminated. Thus, Fig. 91F demonstrates almost no flow to the brain (other than meningeal vessels) following saturation of the basilar inflow.

Diagnosis

Bilateral internal carotid artery occlusions with the intracranial circulation supplied by the basilar artery.

Discussion

This case illustrates the value of saturation pulses in time-of-flight angiography for verifying directionality of flow. Although one can assume that the intracranial circulation is from the basilar system, given the original MR angiographic data, the saturation of signal from the basilar system and resultant nonvisualization of the flow-related enhancement in the remainder of the circulation proves the point. Such saturation pulses can be judiciously employed in various individual vascular distributions for determining relative contribution to flow.

References

1. Edelman RR, Mattle HP, et al. Magnetic resonance imaging of flow dynamics in the circle of Willis. *Stroke* 1990;21:56–65.
2. Felmlee JP, Ehman RL. Spatial presaturation: a method for suppressing flow artifacts and improving depiction of vascular anatomy in MR imaging. *Radiology* 1987;164:559–564.
3. Edelman R, Wendt KU, et al. Intracerebral arteriovenous malformations: evaluation with selective MR angiography and venography. *Radiology* 1989;173:831–837.

Submitted by: Michael Brant-Zawadzki, M.D., F.A.C.R., Hoag Memorial Hospital, Newport Beach, California; Michael Brant-Zawadzki, M.D., F.A.C.R., Senior Editor.

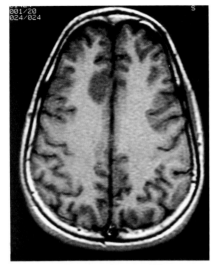

FIG. 92A. SE 500/20.

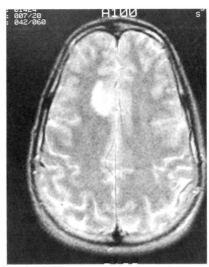

FIG. 92B. SE 2500/80.

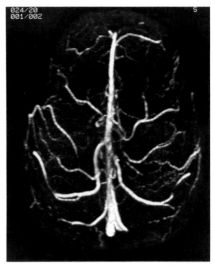

FIG. 92C. 2D TOF MRA (45/9/60°) post-processed 2D collapsed reprojections.

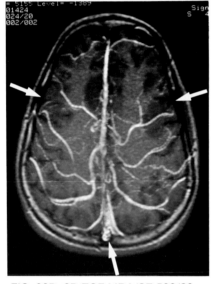

FIG. 92D. 2D TOF MRA/SE 500/20.

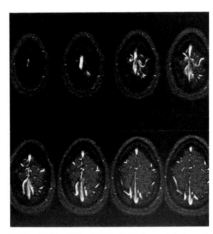

FIG. 92E. 2D TOF MRA axial input slices.

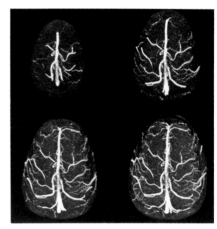

FIG. 92F. 2D TOF MRA post-processed multi-level 2D collapsed reprojections.

Clinical History

A 17-year-old male involved in a motor vehicle accident.

Findings

T1-weighted image (Fig. 92A) shows a right frontal subcortical lesion isointense to surrounding cortical gray matter. T2-weighted images (Fig. 92B) demonstrate that the lesion has hyperintense signal relative to overlying gray matter. There was no definite mass effect and no contrast enhancement. Computed tomography showed a low attenuating mass without hemorrhage.

The 2D time-of-flight (TOF) magnetic resonance angiography (MRA) 2D collapsed image (Fig. 92C) displays preoperatively the cortical venous anatomy. Superimposition of the spin-echo image onto the cortical venous map (Fig. 92D) precisely demonstrates the relationship of the superficial cortical veins to the underlying lesion. The underlying cortical venous anatomy at the level of the coronal sutures can also be discerned (Fig. 92D, *arrowheads*) and the coronal sutures can easily be localized by the neurosurgeon using external palpation.

Diagnosis

Preoperative topographic cortical venous mapping.

Discussion

Several MRA acquisition techniques exist to image the vasculature of the brain. Because of its greater sensitivity to slow flow (1) 2D TOF MRA lends itself best to imaging the cortical venous system. Multiple 1.5-mm input images are generated from the vertex of the head (Fig. 92E) through the level of the lesion. Using a maximum intensity pixel (MIP) postprocessing algorithm consecutive 2D collapsed reprojection images can be generated (Fig. 92F). The postprocessed image incorporating the MRA images to the level of the lesion (Fig. 92F, *lower left image*) can be easily superimposed onto the spin-echo image (Fig. 92D), which also provides a reference for the anatomical visualization of the coronal suture. Fidelity for accurate localization can be confirmed when the flow-related enhancement of the superior sagittal sinus (SSS) in the 2D collapsed MRA (Fig. 92C, *arrow*) precisely superimposes over the flow void of the SSS on the spin-echo image (Fig. 92D, *arrow*).

Reference

1. Keller PJ, Drayer BP, Fram EK, et al. MR angiography with two-dimensional acquisition and three dimensional display—work in progress. *Radiology* 1989;173:527–532.

Submitted by: Orest B. Boyko, M.D., Ph.D., Duke University Medical Center, Durham, North Carolina; Michael Brant-Zawadzki, M.D., F.A.C.R., Senior Editor.

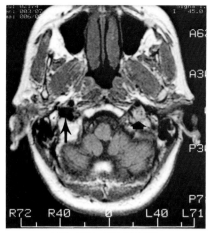

FIG. 93A. SE 500/20.

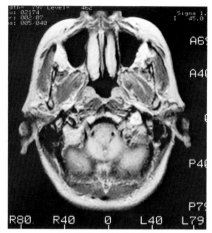

FIG. 93B. SE 2100/30.

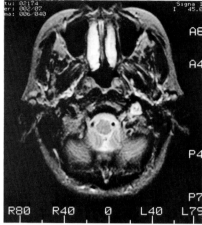

FIG. 93C. SE 2100/80.

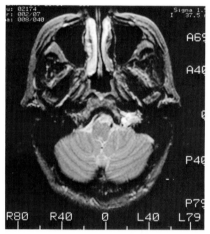

FIG. 93D. SE 2100/80.

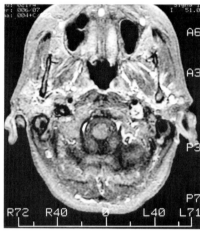

FIG. 93E. Contrast SE 500/20.

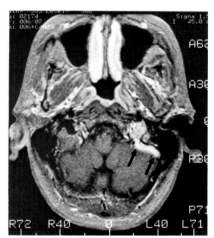

FIG. 93F. Contrast SE 500/20.

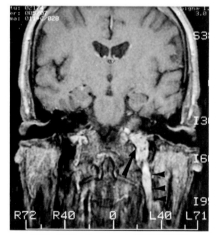

FIG. 93G. Contrast SE 600/20.

Clinical History

A 64-year-old female with left-sided cranial nerves IX, X, XI, and XII deficits.

Findings

Axial T1-weighted image shows signal intensity in the dilated left jugular vein (Fig. 93A, *arrowhead*) as compared with the right, which has a flow void (Fig. 93A, *arrow*). Intermediate and T2-weighted images (Fig. 93B and C) reveal the left jugular vein to have high signal intensity. The hyperintense signal extends to the jugular foramen on the left (Fig. 93D) as seen on a T2-weighted image. There is invasion into the left hypoglossal canal. Contrast-enhanced T1-weighted images with fat suppression saturation pulse reveal the enhancing jugular vein mass (Fig. 93E) with proximal slow flow or enhancing thrombus in the left sigmoid/transverse sinus (Fig. 93F, *arrows*). The mass is visualized on T1-weighted coronal image giving a "salt and pepper" appearance (Fig. 93G, *arrow*) with contrast enhancement in the distal jugular vein representing slow flow or thrombus (Fig. 93G, *arrowheads*).

Diagnosis

Left glomus jugular tumor (paraganglioma).

Discussion

The lack of a homogeneous short T1 signal in the left jugular vein makes spontaneous venous thrombosis unlikely. A meningioma would not tend to have as bright a signal intensity on T2-weighted images as in this case and a neuroma would not have a salt and pepper appearance, which results from the prominent dilated vascular channels intrinsic to a paraganglioma.

The jugular foramen is bounded anterolaterally by the petrous bone and posteromedially by the occipital bone. The two compartments of the jugular foramen are the pars nervosa (cranial nerve IX, glossopharyngeal) and pars vascularis (cranial nerves X and XI, vagus and spiral accessory). The glossopharyngeal nerve gives a peripheral tympanic branch (Jacobson's nerve; glomus tympanicum) and the vagus nerve gives off a postauricular branch (Arnold's nerve; glomus vagale).

References

1. Lo WWM, Solti-Bohman LG. High-resolution CT of the jugular foramen: anatomy and vascular variants and anomalies. *Radiology* 1984;150:743–747.
2. Lo WWM, Solti-Bohman LG, Lambert PR. High-resolution CT in the evaluation of glomus tumors of the temporal bone. *Radiology* 1984;150:737–742.
3. Daniels DL, Czervionke LF, Pech P, et al. Gradient recalled echo MR imaging of the jugular foramen. *AJNR* 1988;9:675–679.
4. Som PM, Sacher M, Stollman AI, et al. Common tumors of the parapharyngeal space: refined imaging diagnosis. *Radiology* 1988;169:81–85.

Submitted by: Orest B. Boyko, M.D., Ph.D., Duke University Medical Center, Durham, North Carolina; Michael Brant-Zawadzki, M.D., F.A.C.R., Senior Editor.

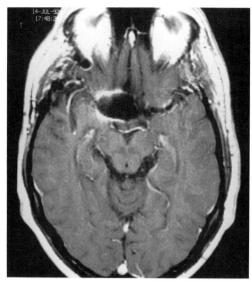

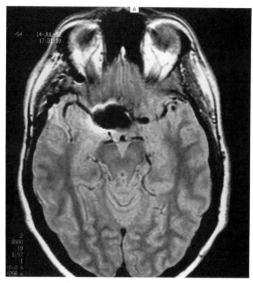

FIG. 94A. Postcontrast axial SE 720/22.

FIG. 94B. Axial SE 3500/19.

Clinical History

A 34-year-old male with recurrent headaches and prior aneurysm surgery.

Findings

The postcontrast T1-weighted axial image (Fig. 94A) shows a large signal void region centered on the right internal carotid artery bifurcation. Note the artifactual rim of high signal intensity surrounding the low signal void. The branches of the middle cerebral artery in the horizontal cistern are identified. The T2-weighted (first echo) axial image (Fig. 94B) demonstrates similar findings. The 3D time-of-flight angiogram (Fig. 94C) shows apparent lack of flow in the distal internal carotid artery and proximal middle cerebral artery M-1 segment. The distal middle cerebral artery M-1 segment is faintly visualized. The standard radiograph of the skull (Fig. 94D) clearly depicts the two aneurysm clips.

Diagnosis

Ferromagnetic artifact due to aneurysm clip with patency of distal vasculature.

Discussion

Aneurysm clipping is a relative contraindication to magnetic resonance imaging. However, the newer generation of clips are MRI safe. Specifically, the titanium type of clip (as in this case) will not be deflected in the magnetic field. Nevertheless, it does induce significant magnetic field inhomogeneity in its vicinity accounting for the artifact depicted here. This magnetic field inhomogeneity may artifactually produce the appearance of vascular occlusion. The observation that the distal vessels are patent on the conventional spin-echo images is essential to appreciating the fact that vessel patency beyond the aneurysm clip is maintained.

References

1. Shellock FG, Crues JV. High-field strength MR imaging and metallic biomedical implants: an ex vivo evaluation of deflection forces. *AJR* 1988;151:389–392.
2. Becker BL, Norfray JF, et al. MR imaging in patients with intracranial aneurysm clips. *AJNR* 1988;9:885–889.
3. Shellock FG, Curtis JS. MR imaging and biomedical implants, materials, and devices: an updated review. *Radiology* 1991;80:541–550.

Submitted by: Michael Brant-Zawadzki, M.D., F.A.C.R., Hoag Memorial Hospital, Newport Beach, California; Michael Brant-Zawadzki, M.D., F.A.C.R., Senior Editor.

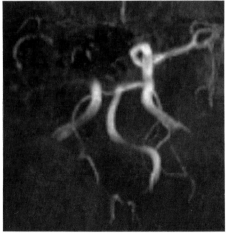

FIG. 94C. MRA 3D TDF (FISP) 30/7/20°.

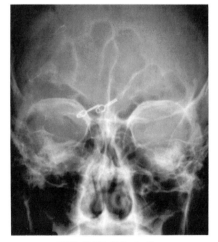

FIG. 94D. PA skull.

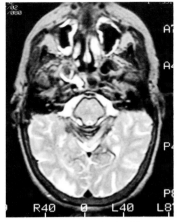 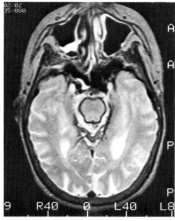 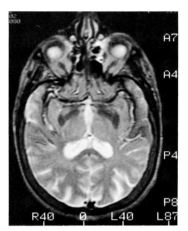

FIG. 95A. SE 2500/80.   FIG. 95B. SE 2500/80.   FIG. 95C. SE 2500/80.

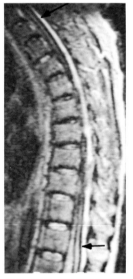 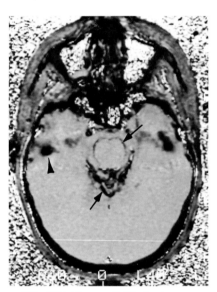

FIG. 95D. SE 2000/70.   FIG. 95E. Susceptibility brain map.

Clinical History

A 64-year-old female presented with progressive deafness and cerebellar ataxia.

Findings

Axial T2-weighted images (Figs. 95A–C) show marked hypointense signal (T2 shortening) throughout the subarachnoid space, extending into the sylvian fissures. Subarachnoid hypointense signal extended into the cervical and thoracic (Fig. 95D, *arrow*) spine. Postprocessed T2 prime susceptibility brain map highlights the areas of magnetic field inhomogeneity (regions of hypointense T2 signal) in the brain from hemosiderin as areas of black (Fig. 95E, *arrows*). Regions without magnetic field inhomogeneity have neutral gray scale. Note the presence of artifactual (nonhemosiderin) areas of magnetic field inhomogeneity [created by brain/bone (petrous ridge) interface] (Fig. 95E, *arrowhead*). There was no associated contrast enhancement of the subarachnoid space.

Diagnosis

Idiopathic superficial siderosis of the central nervous system.

Discussion

Superficial siderosis (SS) consists of hemosiderin deposition in the leptomeninges and subpial tissue surrounding the spinal cord, brain, and cranial nerves (1,2). On T2-weighted MR images areas containing paramagnetic hemosiderin create local magnetic field gradients, which are associated with signal loss due to dephasing of diffusing water protons (1). Patients with SS present with progressive cerebellar ataxia, neurosensory hearing loss, and myelopathy. The cerebellar cortex and eighth cranial nerves appear to have selective vulnerability. In this case hypointense signal of the eighth nerve was difficult to appreciate but positive findings on MR imaging have been reported (1).

Underlying causes for the siderosis include chronic bleeding from small arteriovenous malformations, chronic subdural hematoma, and distal spinal cord (conus) ependymoma (1,2). The cause for posthemorrhage in this case was not identified.

References

1. Gomori JM, Grossman RI, Bilaniuk L, et al. High-field MR imaging of superficial siderosis of the central nervous system. *J Comput Assist Tomogr* 1985;9:972–975.
2. Koepper AH, Dentinger MP. Brain hemosiderin and superficial siderosis of the central nervous system. *J Neuropathol Exp Neurol* 1988;47:249–270.

Submitted by: Orest B. Boyko, M.D., Ph.D., Duke University Medical Center, Durham, North Carolina; Michael Brant-Zawadzki, M.D., F.A.C.R., Senior Editor.

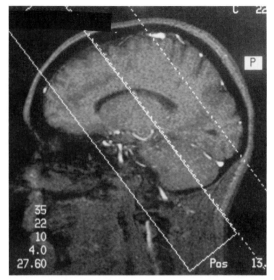

FIG. 96A. Scout image with graphic prescription.

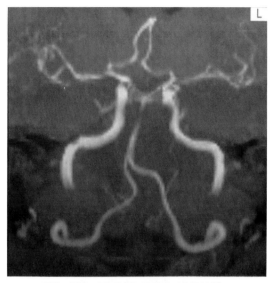

FIG. 96B. 3D TOF (FISP) 40/7/15°.

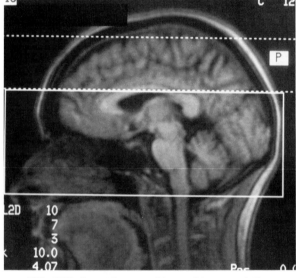

FIG. 96C. Scout image with graphic prescription.

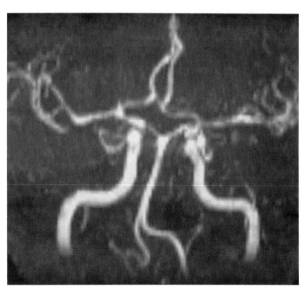

FIG. 96D. 3D TOF (FISP) 40/7/15°.

Clinical History

A 50-year-old female with visual disturbance.

Findings

The initial 3D time-of-flight MR angiogram was obtained for vertebral basilar evaluation, utilizing an angled slab as shown in Fig. 96A. Note the saturation band (*dashed lines*) above the slab to eliminate venous inflow. The resulting maximum intensity projection (Fig. 96B) suggests a distal basilar occlusive lesion. When the study was repeated (Fig. 96C), an axial slab was utilized instead. Note the difference in the appearance of the basilar artery on the resulting projections (Fig. 96D).

Diagnosis

Dephasing artifacts simulating basilar occlusive disease.

Discussion

Close inspection of the oblique coronal partition images at the level of the distal basilar artery (Fig. 96E) reveals a dark band crossing the basilar artery close to its bifurcation distally. The partition image from the axial slab (Fig. 96F) reveals that this is an artifact secondary to magnetic susceptibility effects from the well-aerated sphenoid sinus and dense cortex of the clivus immediately anterior to the basilar artery. This case illustrates the importance of verifying abnormalities on the projection images by reference to the original partitions. Also, elimination of the artifact was made possible by orienting the slab perpendicular to the direction of flow, thus improving inflow of unsaturated spins. The additional dephasing from magnetic susceptibility effects shown in Fig. 96E is overcome by proper optimization of time-of-flight inflow effects.

References

1. Ruggieri PM, Laub GA, et al. Intracranial circulation: pulse sequence considerations in three-dimensional (volume) MR angiography. *Radiology* 1989;171:785–791.
2. Turski P, Bernstein M, Boyko OB, et al. *Vascular magnetic resonance imaging.* GE Medical Systems Application Guide, Milwaukee, WI, 1990.

Submitted by: Michael Brant-Zawadzki, M.D., F.A.C.R., Hoag Memorial Hospital, Newport Beach, California; Michael Brant-Zawadzki, M.D., F.A.C.R., Senior Editor.

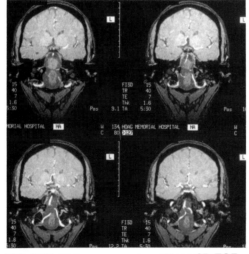

FIG. 96E. Oblique coronal partitions 3D TOF (FISP) 40/7/15°.

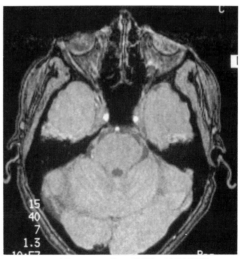

FIG. 96F. 3D TOF (FISP) 40/7/15°.

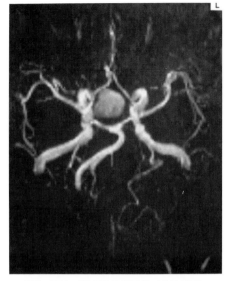

FIG. 97A. 3D TOF (FISP) 40/7/15°.

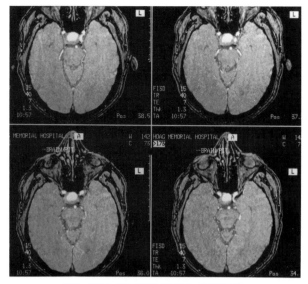

FIG. 97B. 3D TOF (FISP) 40/7/15°.

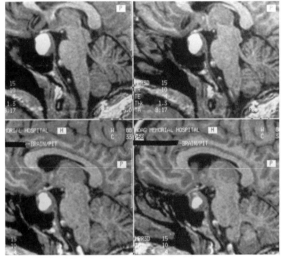

FIG. 97C. MP RAGE sagittal 10/4/15°.

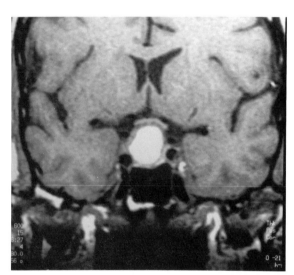

FIG. 97D. SE coronal 600/15°.

Clinical History

A 51-year-old male with visual symptoms.

Findings

The 3D time-of-flight magnetic resonance angiogram (MRA) (Fig. 97A) demonstrates the vertebral basilar and carotid circulations on a base view. In the center of the circle of Willis, a high signal structure is apparent with well-circumscribed borders. The partitions (Fig. 97B) demonstrate the structure as centered on the pituitary fossa. The T1-weighted sagittal (Fig. 97C) and coronal (Fig. 97D) images indicate that the lesion is a high signal mass within the pituitary fossa, which at surgery proved to be a hemorrhagic pituitary macroadenoma.

Diagnosis

Hemorrhagic pituitary macroadenoma.

Discussion

This case demonstrates the nonspecificity of the maximum intensity pixel (MIP) projection algorithm. Any high signal structure of sufficient intensity will be selected by this algorithm just as the high signal vascular channels are. Therefore, these structures may simulate vessels or their pathology (such as aneurysm in this case). Careful evaluation of Fig. 97A reveals that there is no definite contact point for the structure in the pituitary fossa with the surrounding vessels. Nevertheless, this can be a very difficult distinction on the basis of the MRA study alone. Again, correlation with conventional spin-echo images makes the diagnosis easy. Phase contrast angiography would not produce this artifact, as this technique relies more specifically on the velocity of moving spins for the generation of signal intensity. Therefore, stationary high signal structures would not be depicted on phase contrast angiography in similar fashion to blood vessels. Other causes of high signal that may artifactually simulate or obscure vessels include fat (see Case 98), and magnetic susceptibility or "ringing artifacts."

References

1. Anderson CM, Saloner D. Artifacts in maximum-intensity-projection display of MR angiograms. *AJR* 1990;154:623–629.
2. Masaryk TJ, Ross JS. MR angiography: clinical applications. In: Atlas SW, ed. *Magnetic resonance imaging of the brain and spine.* New York: Raven Press, 1991;1079–1097.
3. Huston J, Rufenacht DA, et al. Intracranial aneurysms and vascular malformations: comparison of time-of-flight and phase-contrast MR angiography. *Radiology* 1991;181:721–730.

Submitted by: Michael Brant-Zawadzki, M.D., F.A.C.R., Hoag Memorial Hospital, Newport Beach, California; Michael Brant-Zawadzki, M.D., F.A.C.R., Senior Editor.

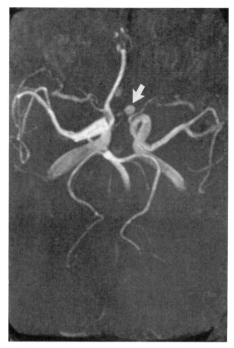

FIG. 98A. 3D TOF (FISP) 33/8/20°.

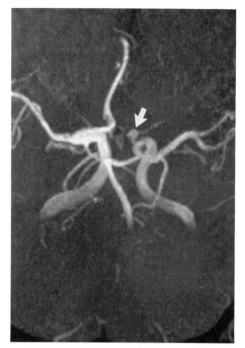

FIG. 98B. 3D TOF (FISP) 33/8/20°.

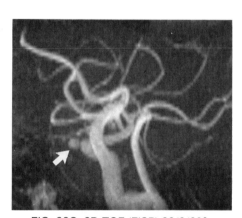

FIG. 98C. 3D TOF (FISP) 33/8/20°.

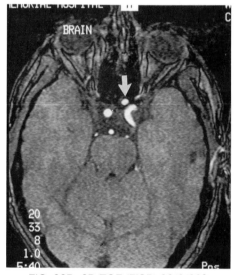

FIG. 98D. 3D TOF (FISP) 33/8/20°.

Clinical History

A 50-year-old male, status postresection of a cavernous sinus meningioma, now presents with vague dizziness.

Findings

The MR angiogram (Figs. 98A–C) demonstrates a small high signal structure suggesting an aneurysm (*arrows*) at the junction of the left internal carotid artery and hypoplastic A-1 segment. These various rotations (Figs. 98A–C) show the constant relationship of this structure to the loop of the periclinoid carotid artery. The partition image (Fig. 98D) also suggests a possible aneurysm (*arrow*).

Diagnosis

Iatrogenically placed fat-simulating aneurysm.

Discussion

The T1-weighted sagittal images (Fig. 98E and F) verify the fat packing in the sphenoid sinus, extending up to the left periclinoid level (*arrow*). The maximum intensity projection algorithm incorrectly "assumed" that this was a vascular structure. This case again demonstrates the nonspecificity of the maximum intensity projection method for selecting bright pixels and placing them in the image. The breakdown products of blood is another entity that can produce such a phenomenon, as can the "bright spot" of the pars nervosa.

Reference

1. Anderson CM, Saloner D. Artifacts in maximum-intensity-projection display of MR angiograms. *AJR* 1990;154:623–629.

Submitted by: Michael Brant-Zawadzki, M.D., F.A.C.R., Hoag Memorial Hospital, Newport Beach, California; Michael Brant-Zawadzki, M.D., F.A.C.R., Senior Editor.

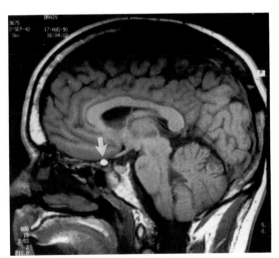

FIG. 98E. Sagittal SE 600/15.

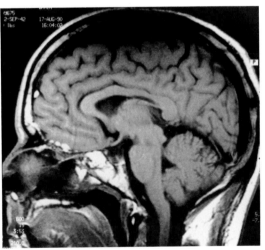

FIG. 98F. Sagittal SE 600/15.

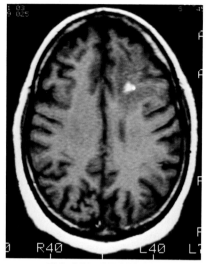

FIG. 99A. SE 500/20.

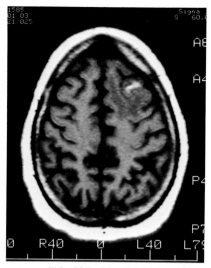

FIG. 99B. SE 500/20.

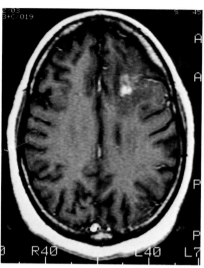

FIG. 99C. SE 500/20 with contrast.

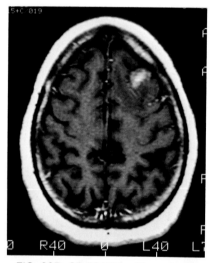

FIG. 99D. SE 500/20 with contrast.

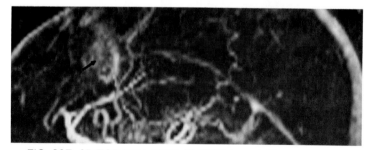

FIG. 99E. 3D TOF MRA (GRE 40/7/20) lateral 3D reprojection.

Clinical History

A 52-year-old male with new seizure onset 3 days previously.

Findings

Axial T1-weighted images show a left frontal lobe hypointense lesion with hyperintense signal indicating hemorrhage (methemoglobin) (Fig. 99A and B). There is minimal surrounding enhancement on T1-weighted images after gadolinium (Gd)-DTPA administration (Fig. 99C and D). The 3D time-of-flight (TOF) magnetic resonance angiography (MRA) 3D reprojection images show bright signal in the left frontal lobe suggesting flow-related enhancement (FRE) (Figs. 99E and F, *arrows*).

Diagnosis

Left frontal lobe hematoma mimicking flow on MRA.

Discussion

The 3D TOF MRA is not sensitive to imaging cerebral veins partly due to the slower flow present in veins compared to arteries becoming saturated in the imaging volume. Intravenous administration of Gd-DTPA promotes better visualization of veins because of the marked change in relaxation times of the venous blood compared to surrounding brain, allowing for a more rapid recovery of longitudinal magnetization (1).

As this case reiterates the presence of areas of shorter T1 in the brain due to paramagnetic effect of methemoglobin and the entrance of Gd-DTPA because of blood-brain barrier disruption can lead to hyperintense signal on MRA, which could be mistaken for FRE and a vascular lesion. Referring back to spin-echo images and identifying methemoglobin ensures proper interpretation.

Reference

1. Chakares DW, Schmalbrock P, Brogan M, et al. Normal venous anatomy of the brain: demonstration with gadopentetate dimeglumine in enhanced 3-D MR angiography. *AJNR* 1990;11:1107–1118.

Submitted by: Orest B. Boyko, M.D., Ph.D., Duke University Medical Center, Durham, North Carolina; Michael Brant-Zawadzki, M.D., F.A.C.R., Senior Editor.

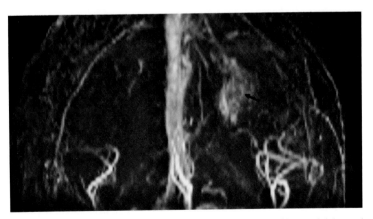

FIG. 99F. 3D TOF MRA (GRE 40/7/20; TR/TE/Deg flip angle) lateral 3D reprojection.

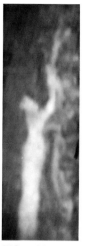
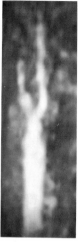
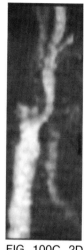
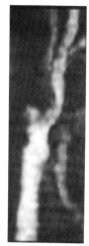

FIG. 100A. 3D TOF MRA, 60/8.

FIG. 100B. 3D TOF MRA, 60/8.

FIG. 100C. 2D TOF MRA, 50/9.

FIG. 100D. 2D TOF MRA, 50/9.

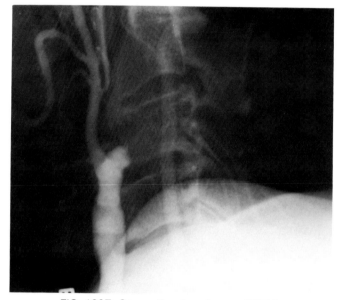

FIG. 100E. Conventional angiogram RCCA.

Clinical History

A 64-year-old male with history of atherosclerotic disease.

Findings

The 3D time-of-flight (TOF) magnetic resonance angiography (MRA) 3D reprojections show the proximal right internal carotid artery (RICA) ending in a stump (Figs. 100A and B). There is no distal flow-related enhancement (FRE) in the ICA, indicating that this is a complete occlusion. The 2D time-of-flight MRA 3D reprojections also demonstrate the occlusion (Figs. 100C and D). Note that on a given rotational projection (Fig. 100B) the FRE of an overlapping vessel can project directly over the occluded stump (Fig. 100D).

Conventional right common carotid artery (CCA) angiogram shows the occluded stump of the RICA (Fig. 100E).

Diagnosis

Asymptomatic occlusion RICA from atherosclerotic disease.

Discussion

Lack of multiple 3D reprojections from acquired MRA partition images can lead to a pitfall of misinterpretation of carotid arteries as not being occluded (1). The ability of carotid MRA to distinguish slow flow states of the "string sign" from complete occlusions is still yet to be determined (2).

References

1. Litt AW, Eidelman EM, Pinto RS, et al. Diagnosis of carotid artery stenosis: comparison of 2DFT time-of-flight MR angiography with contrast angiography in 50 patients. *AJNR* 1991;12:149–154.
2. Masaryk AM, Ross JS, DiCello MC, et al. 3DFT MR angiography of the carotid bifurcation: potential and limitations as a screening examination. *Radiology* 1991;179:797–804.

Submitted by: Orest B. Boyko, M.D., Ph.D., Duke University Medical Center, Durham, North Carolina; Michael Brant-Zawadzki, M.D., F.A.C.R., Senior Editor.

245